# This Beekeeping log Book

## Belongs to
_____

## DEDICATION

This Beekeeping Log Book is dedicated to all the beekeepers out there who love working with bees.

You are my inspiration for producing books and I'm honored to be a part of keeping all of your important information and ideas organized all in one easy to find spot.

# How to use this Beekeeping Log Book:

This ultimate beekeeping log notebook is a perfect way to track and record all your beekeeping activities. This unique Beekeeper's Journal is a great way to keep all of your important information all in one easy to find spot.

Each interior page includes prompts and space to record the following:

1. Colony Name - Write the name of the colony.

2. Date - Use the box provided to write in the date.

3. Weather Conditions - Stay on task using this space to record weather from sunny to rainy conditions.

4. Inspection - Rate the bee hive from 1-6 upon inspection.

5. Hive Number - Use the box to check mark the bee hive.

6. Productivity/Reproduction - Stay on task using the boxes for amount of honey, general population, amount of brood, and amount of space.

7. Behavior and Activities - Write the usual entering and ending activities, calm behavior when opening hive, bees bringing to hive, signs of robbery among the bees.

8. Health Status - Checklist if the bees seem weak or lazy, high amount of dead bees, queen bee is present, if she is identifiable, any infestation by ants, wax moth or any negative odor noted.

If you are new to beekeeping or have been at it for a while, this cute beekeeping journal is a must have! Can make a great useful gift for anyone that loves the hobby of beekeeping!

Have Fun!

| COLONY NAME | | WEATHER CONDITIONS | |
|---|---|---|---|
| DATE | | 🌡 ___ ☀ ⛅ 🌧 ⛈ ❄ | |
| TIME | | 🚩 ___ ☐ ☐ ☐ ☐ ☐ | |

## INSPECTION

| HIVE NUMBER | 1 | 2 | 3 | 4 | 5 | 6 |
|---|---|---|---|---|---|---|

### PRODUCTIVITY & REPRODUCTION

| | | | | | | |
|---|---|---|---|---|---|---|
| AMOUNT OF HONEY | | | | | | |
| GENERAL POPULATION | | | | | | |
| AMOUNT OF BROOD | | | | | | |
| AMOUNT OF SPACE | | | | | | |

### BEHAVIOUR & ACTIVITIES

| | | | | | | |
|---|---|---|---|---|---|---|
| USUAL ENTERING AND EXITING ACTIVITY? | | | | | | |
| CALM BEHAVIOUR WHEN OPENING HIVE? | | | | | | |
| BEES BRINGING POLLEN INTO HIVE? | | | | | | |
| SIGNS OF ROBBERY AMONG THE BEES? | | | | | | |

### HEALTH STATUS

| | | | | | | |
|---|---|---|---|---|---|---|
| BEES SEEM WEAK OR LAZY? | | | | | | |
| HIGH AMOUNT OF DEAD BEES? | | | | | | |
| QUEEN BEE IS PRESENT / IDENTIFIABLE? | | | | | | |
| INFESTATION BY ANTS / ANTS PRESENT? | | | | | | |
| INFESTATION BY WAX MOTH / WAX MOTH PRESENT? | | | | | | |
| NEGATIVE ODOUR NOTICEABLE? | | | | | | |

| | COLONY NAME |
|---|---|
| | DATE |
| | TIME |

**WEATHER CONDITIONS**

🌡️ ____ ☀️ ⛅ 🌧️ ⛈️ ❄️
🚩 ____ ☐ ☐ ☐ ☐ ☐

## INSPECTION

| HIVE NUMBER | ① | ② | ③ | ④ | ⑤ | ⑥ |
|---|---|---|---|---|---|---|

## PRODUCTIVITY & REPRODUCTION

| | | | | | | |
|---|---|---|---|---|---|---|
| AMOUNT OF HONEY | | | | | | |
| GENERAL POPULATION | | | | | | |
| AMOUNT OF BROOD | | | | | | |
| AMOUNT OF SPACE | | | | | | |

## BEHAVIOUR & ACTIVITIES

| | | | | | | |
|---|---|---|---|---|---|---|
| USUAL ENTERING AND EXITING ACTIVITY? | | | | | | |
| CALM BEHAVIOUR WHEN OPENING HIVE? | | | | | | |
| BEES BRINGING POLLEN INTO HIVE? | | | | | | |
| SIGNS OF ROBBERY AMONG THE BEES? | | | | | | |

## HEALTH STATUS

| | | | | | | |
|---|---|---|---|---|---|---|
| BEES SEEM WEAK OR LAZY? | | | | | | |
| HIGH AMOUNT OF DEAD BEES? | | | | | | |
| QUEEN BEE IS PRESENT / IDENTIFIABLE? | | | | | | |
| INFESTATION BY ANTS / ANTS PRESENT? | | | | | | |
| INFESTATION BY WAX MOTH / WAX MOTH PRESENT? | | | | | | |
| NEGATIVE ODOUR NOTICEABLE? | | | | | | |

| COLONY NAME | |
|---|---|
| DATE | |
| TIME | |

| WEATHER CONDITIONS | | | | | |
|---|---|---|---|---|---|
| 🌡 ___ | ☀ | ⛅ | 🌧 | ⛈ | ❄ |
| 🚩 ___ | ☐ | ☐ | ☐ | ☐ | ☐ |

## INSPECTION

| HIVE NUMBER | 1 | 2 | 3 | 4 | 5 | 6 |
|---|---|---|---|---|---|---|

### PRODUCTIVITY & REPRODUCTION

| | | | | | | |
|---|---|---|---|---|---|---|
| AMOUNT OF HONEY | | | | | | |
| GENERAL POPULATION | | | | | | |
| AMOUNT OF BROOD | | | | | | |
| AMOUNT OF SPACE | | | | | | |

### BEHAVIOUR & ACTIVITIES

| | | | | | | |
|---|---|---|---|---|---|---|
| USUAL ENTERING AND EXITING ACTIVITY? | | | | | | |
| CALM BEHAVIOUR WHEN OPENING HIVE? | | | | | | |
| BEES BRINGING POLLEN INTO HIVE? | | | | | | |
| SIGNS OF ROBBERY AMONG THE BEES? | | | | | | |

### HEALTH STATUS

| | | | | | | |
|---|---|---|---|---|---|---|
| BEES SEEM WEAK OR LAZY? | | | | | | |
| HIGH AMOUNT OF DEAD BEES? | | | | | | |
| QUEEN BEE IS PRESENT / IDENTIFIABLE? | | | | | | |
| INFESTATION BY ANTS / ANTS PRESENT? | | | | | | |
| INFESTATION BY WAX MOTH / WAX MOTH PRESENT? | | | | | | |
| NEGATIVE ODOUR NOTICEABLE? | | | | | | |

| COLONY NAME | |
|---|---|
| DATE | |
| TIME | |

## WEATHER CONDITIONS

🌡️ _____   ☀️ ⛅ 🌧️ ⛈️ ❄️
🚩 _____   ☐  ☐  ☐  ☐  ☐

## INSPECTION

| HIVE NUMBER | ① | ② | ③ | ④ | ⑤ | ⑥ |
|---|---|---|---|---|---|---|

## PRODUCTIVITY & REPRODUCTION

| | | | | | | |
|---|---|---|---|---|---|---|
| AMOUNT OF HONEY | | | | | | |
| GENERAL POPULATION | | | | | | |
| AMOUNT OF BROOD | | | | | | |
| AMOUNT OF SPACE | | | | | | |

## BEHAVIOUR & ACTIVITIES

| | | | | | | |
|---|---|---|---|---|---|---|
| USUAL ENTERING AND EXITING ACTIVITY? | | | | | | |
| CALM BEHAVIOUR WHEN OPENING HIVE? | | | | | | |
| BEES BRINGING POLLEN INTO HIVE? | | | | | | |
| SIGNS OF ROBBERY AMONG THE BEES? | | | | | | |

## HEALTH STATUS

| | | | | | | |
|---|---|---|---|---|---|---|
| BEES SEEM WEAK OR LAZY? | | | | | | |
| HIGH AMOUNT OF DEAD BEES? | | | | | | |
| QUEEN BEE IS PRESENT / IDENTIFIABLE? | | | | | | |
| INFESTATION BY ANTS / ANTS PRESENT? | | | | | | |
| INFESTATION BY WAX MOTH / WAX MOTH PRESENT? | | | | | | |
| NEGATIVE ODOUR NOTICEABLE? | | | | | | |

|  | COLONY NAME |
|--|--|
|  | DATE |
|  | TIME |

**WEATHER CONDITIONS**

🌡 ——   ☀ ⛅ 🌧 ⛈ ❄

🚩 ——   ☐ ☐ ☐ ☐ ☐

## INSPECTION

| HIVE NUMBER | ① | ② | ③ | ④ | ⑤ | ⑥ |
|---|---|---|---|---|---|---|

## PRODUCTIVITY & REPRODUCTION

| | | | | | | |
|---|---|---|---|---|---|---|
| AMOUNT OF HONEY | | | | | | |
| GENERAL POPULATION | | | | | | |
| AMOUNT OF BROOD | | | | | | |
| AMOUNT OF SPACE | | | | | | |

## BEHAVIOUR & ACTIVITIES

| | | | | | | |
|---|---|---|---|---|---|---|
| USUAL ENTERING AND EXITING ACTIVITY? | | | | | | |
| CALM BEHAVIOUR WHEN OPENING HIVE? | | | | | | |
| BEES BRINGING POLLEN INTO HIVE? | | | | | | |
| SIGNS OF ROBBERY AMONG THE BEES? | | | | | | |

## HEALTH STATUS

| | | | | | | |
|---|---|---|---|---|---|---|
| BEES SEEM WEAK OR LAZY? | | | | | | |
| HIGH AMOUNT OF DEAD BEES? | | | | | | |
| QUEEN BEE IS PRESENT / IDENTIFIABLE? | | | | | | |
| INFESTATION BY ANTS / ANTS PRESENT? | | | | | | |
| INFESTATION BY WAX MOTH / WAX MOTH PRESENT? | | | | | | |
| NEGATIVE ODOUR NOTICEABLE? | | | | | | |

|  | COLONY NAME |
|---|---|
|  | DATE |
|  | TIME |

**WEATHER CONDITIONS**

| 🌡 | ___ | ☀ | ⛅ | 🌧 | ⛈ | ❄ |
|---|---|---|---|---|---|---|
| 🚩 | ___ | ☐ | ☐ | ☐ | ☐ | ☐ |

## INSPECTION

| HIVE NUMBER | ① | ② | ③ | ④ | ⑤ | ⑥ |
|---|---|---|---|---|---|---|

## PRODUCTIVITY & REPRODUCTION

| | | | | | | |
|---|---|---|---|---|---|---|
| AMOUNT OF HONEY | | | | | | |
| GENERAL POPULATION | | | | | | |
| AMOUNT OF BROOD | | | | | | |
| AMOUNT OF SPACE | | | | | | |

## BEHAVIOUR & ACTIVITIES

| | | | | | | |
|---|---|---|---|---|---|---|
| USUAL ENTERING AND EXITING ACTIVITY? | | | | | | |
| CALM BEHAVIOUR WHEN OPENING HIVE? | | | | | | |
| BEES BRINGING POLLEN INTO HIVE? | | | | | | |
| SIGNS OF ROBBERY AMONG THE BEES? | | | | | | |

## HEALTH STATUS

| | | | | | | |
|---|---|---|---|---|---|---|
| BEES SEEM WEAK OR LAZY? | | | | | | |
| HIGH AMOUNT OF DEAD BEES? | | | | | | |
| QUEEN BEE IS PRESENT / IDENTIFIABLE? | | | | | | |
| INFESTATION BY ANTS / ANTS PRESENT? | | | | | | |
| INFESTATION BY WAX MOTH / WAX MOTH PRESENT? | | | | | | |
| NEGATIVE ODOUR NOTICEABLE? | | | | | | |

| COLONY NAME | |
|---|---|
| DATE | |
| TIME | |

## WEATHER CONDITIONS

🌡 _____  ☀ ⛅ 🌧 ⛈ ❄
🚩 _____  ☐ ☐ ☐ ☐ ☐

## INSPECTION

| HIVE NUMBER | ① | ② | ③ | ④ | ⑤ | ⑥ |
|---|---|---|---|---|---|---|

### PRODUCTIVITY & REPRODUCTION

| | | | | | | |
|---|---|---|---|---|---|---|
| AMOUNT OF HONEY | | | | | | |
| GENERAL POPULATION | | | | | | |
| AMOUNT OF BROOD | | | | | | |
| AMOUNT OF SPACE | | | | | | |

### BEHAVIOUR & ACTIVITIES

| | | | | | | |
|---|---|---|---|---|---|---|
| USUAL ENTERING AND EXITING ACTIVITY? | | | | | | |
| CALM BEHAVIOUR WHEN OPENING HIVE? | | | | | | |
| BEES BRINGING POLLEN INTO HIVE? | | | | | | |
| SIGNS OF ROBBERY AMONG THE BEES? | | | | | | |

### HEALTH STATUS

| | | | | | | |
|---|---|---|---|---|---|---|
| BEES SEEM WEAK OR LAZY? | | | | | | |
| HIGH AMOUNT OF DEAD BEES? | | | | | | |
| QUEEN BEE IS PRESENT / IDENTIFIABLE? | | | | | | |
| INFESTATION BY ANTS / ANTS PRESENT? | | | | | | |
| INFESTATION BY WAX MOTH / WAX MOTH PRESENT? | | | | | | |
| NEGATIVE ODOUR NOTICEABLE? | | | | | | |

|  | COLONY NAME |
|---|---|
|  | DATE |
|  | TIME |

## WEATHER CONDITIONS

🌡 _____  ☀ ⛅ 🌧 ⛈ ❄
🚩 _____  ☐ ☐ ☐ ☐ ☐

## INSPECTION

| HIVE NUMBER | ① | ② | ③ | ④ | ⑤ | ⑥ |
|---|---|---|---|---|---|---|

## PRODUCTIVITY & REPRODUCTION

| | | | | | | |
|---|---|---|---|---|---|---|
| AMOUNT OF HONEY | | | | | | |
| GENERAL POPULATION | | | | | | |
| AMOUNT OF BROOD | | | | | | |
| AMOUNT OF SPACE | | | | | | |

## BEHAVIOUR & ACTIVITIES

| | | | | | | |
|---|---|---|---|---|---|---|
| USUAL ENTERING AND EXITING ACTIVITY? | | | | | | |
| CALM BEHAVIOUR WHEN OPENING HIVE? | | | | | | |
| BEES BRINGING POLLEN INTO HIVE? | | | | | | |
| SIGNS OF ROBBERY AMONG THE BEES? | | | | | | |

## HEALTH STATUS

| | | | | | | |
|---|---|---|---|---|---|---|
| BEES SEEM WEAK OR LAZY? | | | | | | |
| HIGH AMOUNT OF DEAD BEES? | | | | | | |
| QUEEN BEE IS PRESENT / IDENTIFIABLE? | | | | | | |
| INFESTATION BY ANTS / ANTS PRESENT? | | | | | | |
| INFESTATION BY WAX MOTH / WAX MOTH PRESENT? | | | | | | |
| NEGATIVE ODOUR NOTICEABLE? | | | | | | |

| COLONY NAME | |
|---|---|
| DATE | |
| TIME | |

**WEATHER CONDITIONS**

🌡 ____  ☀ ☁ 🌦 ⛈ ❄
🚩 ____  ☐ ☐ ☐ ☐ ☐

## INSPECTION

| HIVE NUMBER | 1 | 2 | 3 | 4 | 5 | 6 |
|---|---|---|---|---|---|---|

## PRODUCTIVITY & REPRODUCTION

| | | | | | | |
|---|---|---|---|---|---|---|
| AMOUNT OF HONEY | | | | | | |
| GENERAL POPULATION | | | | | | |
| AMOUNT OF BROOD | | | | | | |
| AMOUNT OF SPACE | | | | | | |

## BEHAVIOUR & ACTIVITIES

| | | | | | | |
|---|---|---|---|---|---|---|
| USUAL ENTERING AND EXITING ACTIVITY? | | | | | | |
| CALM BEHAVIOUR WHEN OPENING HIVE? | | | | | | |
| BEES BRINGING POLLEN INTO HIVE? | | | | | | |
| SIGNS OF ROBBERY AMONG THE BEES? | | | | | | |

## HEALTH STATUS

| | | | | | | |
|---|---|---|---|---|---|---|
| BEES SEEM WEAK OR LAZY? | | | | | | |
| HIGH AMOUNT OF DEAD BEES? | | | | | | |
| QUEEN BEE IS PRESENT / IDENTIFIABLE? | | | | | | |
| INFESTATION BY ANTS / ANTS PRESENT? | | | | | | |
| INFESTATION BY WAX MOTH / WAX MOTH PRESENT? | | | | | | |
| NEGATIVE ODOUR NOTICEABLE? | | | | | | |

|  | COLONY NAME |
|---|---|
|  | DATE |
|  | TIME |

## WEATHER CONDITIONS

🌡 ____   ☀ ☁ 🌦 ⛈ ❄
🚩 ____   ☐ ☐ ☐ ☐ ☐

## INSPECTION

| HIVE NUMBER | ① | ② | ③ | ④ | ⑤ | ⑥ |
|---|---|---|---|---|---|---|

## PRODUCTIVITY & REPRODUCTION

| | | | | | | |
|---|---|---|---|---|---|---|
| AMOUNT OF HONEY | | | | | | |
| GENERAL POPULATION | | | | | | |
| AMOUNT OF BROOD | | | | | | |
| AMOUNT OF SPACE | | | | | | |

## BEHAVIOUR & ACTIVITIES

| | | | | | | |
|---|---|---|---|---|---|---|
| USUAL ENTERING AND EXITING ACTIVITY? | | | | | | |
| CALM BEHAVIOUR WHEN OPENING HIVE? | | | | | | |
| BEES BRINGING POLLEN INTO HIVE? | | | | | | |
| SIGNS OF ROBBERY AMONG THE BEES? | | | | | | |

## HEALTH STATUS

| | | | | | | |
|---|---|---|---|---|---|---|
| BEES SEEM WEAK OR LAZY? | | | | | | |
| HIGH AMOUNT OF DEAD BEES? | | | | | | |
| QUEEN BEE IS PRESENT / IDENTIFIABLE? | | | | | | |
| INFESTATION BY ANTS / ANTS PRESENT? | | | | | | |
| INFESTATION BY WAX MOTH / WAX MOTH PRESENT? | | | | | | |
| NEGATIVE ODOUR NOTICEABLE? | | | | | | |

|  |  |
|---|---|
| 🏠 COLONY NAME | |
| 📅 DATE | |
| 🕐 TIME | |

| WEATHER CONDITIONS |
|---|
| 🌡 ____  ☀️ ⛅ 🌧 ⛈ ❄️ |
| 🚩 ____  ☐ ☐ ☐ ☐ ☐ |

## INSPECTION

| HIVE NUMBER | 1 | 2 | 3 | 4 | 5 | 6 |
|---|---|---|---|---|---|---|

## PRODUCTIVITY & REPRODUCTION

| | | | | | | |
|---|---|---|---|---|---|---|
| AMOUNT OF HONEY | | | | | | |
| GENERAL POPULATION | | | | | | |
| AMOUNT OF BROOD | | | | | | |
| AMOUNT OF SPACE | | | | | | |

## BEHAVIOUR & ACTIVITIES

| | | | | | | |
|---|---|---|---|---|---|---|
| USUAL ENTERING AND EXITING ACTIVITY? | | | | | | |
| CALM BEHAVIOUR WHEN OPENING HIVE? | | | | | | |
| BEES BRINGING POLLEN INTO HIVE? | | | | | | |
| SIGNS OF ROBBERY AMONG THE BEES? | | | | | | |

## HEALTH STATUS

| | | | | | | |
|---|---|---|---|---|---|---|
| BEES SEEM WEAK OR LAZY? | | | | | | |
| HIGH AMOUNT OF DEAD BEES? | | | | | | |
| QUEEN BEE IS PRESENT / IDENTIFIABLE? | | | | | | |
| INFESTATION BY ANTS / ANTS PRESENT? | | | | | | |
| INFESTATION BY WAX MOTH / WAX MOTH PRESENT? | | | | | | |
| NEGATIVE ODOUR NOTICEABLE? | | | | | | |

|  | COLONY NAME |
|---|---|
|  | DATE |
|  | TIME |

**WEATHER CONDITIONS**

| 🌡 | ___ | ☀ | ⛅ | 🌧 | ⛈ | ❄ |
|---|---|---|---|---|---|---|
| 🚩 | ___ | ☐ | ☐ | ☐ | ☐ | ☐ |

## INSPECTION

| HIVE NUMBER | 1 | 2 | 3 | 4 | 5 | 6 |
|---|---|---|---|---|---|---|

## PRODUCTIVITY & REPRODUCTION

| | | | | | | |
|---|---|---|---|---|---|---|
| AMOUNT OF HONEY | | | | | | |
| GENERAL POPULATION | | | | | | |
| AMOUNT OF BROOD | | | | | | |
| AMOUNT OF SPACE | | | | | | |

## BEHAVIOUR & ACTIVITIES

| | | | | | | |
|---|---|---|---|---|---|---|
| USUAL ENTERING AND EXITING ACTIVITY? | | | | | | |
| CALM BEHAVIOUR WHEN OPENING HIVE? | | | | | | |
| BEES BRINGING POLLEN INTO HIVE? | | | | | | |
| SIGNS OF ROBBERY AMONG THE BEES? | | | | | | |

## HEALTH STATUS

| | | | | | | |
|---|---|---|---|---|---|---|
| BEES SEEM WEAK OR LAZY? | | | | | | |
| HIGH AMOUNT OF DEAD BEES? | | | | | | |
| QUEEN BEE IS PRESENT / IDENTIFIABLE? | | | | | | |
| INFESTATION BY ANTS / ANTS PRESENT? | | | | | | |
| INFESTATION BY WAX MOTH / WAX MOTH PRESENT? | | | | | | |
| NEGATIVE ODOUR NOTICEABLE? | | | | | | |

|  | COLONY NAME |
|---|---|
|  | DATE |
|  | TIME |

**WEATHER CONDITIONS**

🌡 ____ ☀ ⛅ 🌧 ⛈ ❄
🚩 ____ ☐ ☐ ☐ ☐ ☐

## INSPECTION

| HIVE NUMBER | 1 | 2 | 3 | 4 | 5 | 6 |
|---|---|---|---|---|---|---|

### PRODUCTIVITY & REPRODUCTION

| | | | | | | |
|---|---|---|---|---|---|---|
| AMOUNT OF HONEY | | | | | | |
| GENERAL POPULATION | | | | | | |
| AMOUNT OF BROOD | | | | | | |
| AMOUNT OF SPACE | | | | | | |

### BEHAVIOUR & ACTIVITIES

| | | | | | | |
|---|---|---|---|---|---|---|
| USUAL ENTERING AND EXITING ACTIVITY? | | | | | | |
| CALM BEHAVIOUR WHEN OPENING HIVE? | | | | | | |
| BEES BRINGING POLLEN INTO HIVE? | | | | | | |
| SIGNS OF ROBBERY AMONG THE BEES? | | | | | | |

### HEALTH STATUS

| | | | | | | |
|---|---|---|---|---|---|---|
| BEES SEEM WEAK OR LAZY? | | | | | | |
| HIGH AMOUNT OF DEAD BEES? | | | | | | |
| QUEEN BEE IS PRESENT / IDENTIFIABLE? | | | | | | |
| INFESTATION BY ANTS / ANTS PRESENT? | | | | | | |
| INFESTATION BY WAX MOTH / WAX MOTH PRESENT? | | | | | | |
| NEGATIVE ODOUR NOTICEABLE? | | | | | | |

|  | COLONY NAME |
|---|---|
|  | DATE |
|  | TIME |

**WEATHER CONDITIONS**

🌡 _____  ☀ ⛅ 🌦 ⛈ ❄
🚩 _____  ☐ ☐ ☐ ☐ ☐

## INSPECTION

| HIVE NUMBER | ① | ② | ③ | ④ | ⑤ | ⑥ |
|---|---|---|---|---|---|---|

## PRODUCTIVITY & REPRODUCTION

| | | | | | | |
|---|---|---|---|---|---|---|
| AMOUNT OF HONEY | | | | | | |
| GENERAL POPULATION | | | | | | |
| AMOUNT OF BROOD | | | | | | |
| AMOUNT OF SPACE | | | | | | |

## BEHAVIOUR & ACTIVITIES

| | | | | | | |
|---|---|---|---|---|---|---|
| USUAL ENTERING AND EXITING ACTIVITY? | | | | | | |
| CALM BEHAVIOUR WHEN OPENING HIVE? | | | | | | |
| BEES BRINGING POLLEN INTO HIVE? | | | | | | |
| SIGNS OF ROBBERY AMONG THE BEES? | | | | | | |

## HEALTH STATUS

| | | | | | | |
|---|---|---|---|---|---|---|
| BEES SEEM WEAK OR LAZY? | | | | | | |
| HIGH AMOUNT OF DEAD BEES? | | | | | | |
| QUEEN BEE IS PRESENT / IDENTIFIABLE? | | | | | | |
| INFESTATION BY ANTS / ANTS PRESENT? | | | | | | |
| INFESTATION BY WAX MOTH / WAX MOTH PRESENT? | | | | | | |
| NEGATIVE ODOUR NOTICEABLE? | | | | | | |

| COLONY NAME | |
|---|---|
| DATE | |
| TIME | |

| WEATHER CONDITIONS | | | | | |
|---|---|---|---|---|---|
| 🌡 ___ | ☀ | ⛅ | 🌧 | ⛈ | ❄ |
| 🚩 ___ | ☐ | ☐ | ☐ | ☐ | ☐ |

## INSPECTION

| HIVE NUMBER | 1 | 2 | 3 | 4 | 5 | 6 |
|---|---|---|---|---|---|---|

## PRODUCTIVITY & REPRODUCTION

| | | | | | | |
|---|---|---|---|---|---|---|
| AMOUNT OF HONEY | | | | | | |
| GENERAL POPULATION | | | | | | |
| AMOUNT OF BROOD | | | | | | |
| AMOUNT OF SPACE | | | | | | |

## BEHAVIOUR & ACTIVITIES

| | | | | | | |
|---|---|---|---|---|---|---|
| USUAL ENTERING AND EXITING ACTIVITY? | | | | | | |
| CALM BEHAVIOUR WHEN OPENING HIVE? | | | | | | |
| BEES BRINGING POLLEN INTO HIVE? | | | | | | |
| SIGNS OF ROBBERY AMONG THE BEES? | | | | | | |

## HEALTH STATUS

| | | | | | | |
|---|---|---|---|---|---|---|
| BEES SEEM WEAK OR LAZY? | | | | | | |
| HIGH AMOUNT OF DEAD BEES? | | | | | | |
| QUEEN BEE IS PRESENT / IDENTIFIABLE? | | | | | | |
| INFESTATION BY ANTS / ANTS PRESENT? | | | | | | |
| INFESTATION BY WAX MOTH / WAX MOTH PRESENT? | | | | | | |
| NEGATIVE ODOUR NOTICEABLE? | | | | | | |

| COLONY NAME | |
|---|---|
| DATE | |
| TIME | |

**WEATHER CONDITIONS**

🌡 _____  ☀  ⛅  🌧  ⛈  ❄
🪭 _____  ☐  ☐  ☐  ☐  ☐

## INSPECTION

| HIVE NUMBER | ① | ② | ③ | ④ | ⑤ | ⑥ |
|---|---|---|---|---|---|---|

### PRODUCTIVITY & REPRODUCTION

| | | | | | | |
|---|---|---|---|---|---|---|
| AMOUNT OF HONEY | | | | | | |
| GENERAL POPULATION | | | | | | |
| AMOUNT OF BROOD | | | | | | |
| AMOUNT OF SPACE | | | | | | |

### BEHAVIOUR & ACTIVITIES

| | | | | | | |
|---|---|---|---|---|---|---|
| USUAL ENTERING AND EXITING ACTIVITY? | | | | | | |
| CALM BEHAVIOUR WHEN OPENING HIVE? | | | | | | |
| BEES BRINGING POLLEN INTO HIVE? | | | | | | |
| SIGNS OF ROBBERY AMONG THE BEES? | | | | | | |

### HEALTH STATUS

| | | | | | | |
|---|---|---|---|---|---|---|
| BEES SEEM WEAK OR LAZY? | | | | | | |
| HIGH AMOUNT OF DEAD BEES? | | | | | | |
| QUEEN BEE IS PRESENT / IDENTIFIABLE? | | | | | | |
| INFESTATION BY ANTS / ANTS PRESENT? | | | | | | |
| INFESTATION BY WAX MOTH / WAX MOTH PRESENT? | | | | | | |
| NEGATIVE ODOUR NOTICEABLE? | | | | | | |

| | COLONY NAME |
|---|---|
| | DATE |
| | TIME |

**WEATHER CONDITIONS**

🌡 _____  ☀ ☁ 🌧 ⛈ ❄
🚩 _____  ☐ ☐ ☐ ☐ ☐

## INSPECTION

| HIVE NUMBER | 1 | 2 | 3 | 4 | 5 | 6 |
|---|---|---|---|---|---|---|

## PRODUCTIVITY & REPRODUCTION

| | | | | | | |
|---|---|---|---|---|---|---|
| AMOUNT OF HONEY | | | | | | |
| GENERAL POPULATION | | | | | | |
| AMOUNT OF BROOD | | | | | | |
| AMOUNT OF SPACE | | | | | | |

## BEHAVIOUR & ACTIVITIES

| | | | | | | |
|---|---|---|---|---|---|---|
| USUAL ENTERING AND EXITING ACTIVITY? | | | | | | |
| CALM BEHAVIOUR WHEN OPENING HIVE? | | | | | | |
| BEES BRINGING POLLEN INTO HIVE? | | | | | | |
| SIGNS OF ROBBERY AMONG THE BEES? | | | | | | |

## HEALTH STATUS

| | | | | | | |
|---|---|---|---|---|---|---|
| BEES SEEM WEAK OR LAZY? | | | | | | |
| HIGH AMOUNT OF DEAD BEES? | | | | | | |
| QUEEN BEE IS PRESENT / IDENTIFIABLE? | | | | | | |
| INFESTATION BY ANTS / ANTS PRESENT? | | | | | | |
| INFESTATION BY WAX MOTH / WAX MOTH PRESENT? | | | | | | |
| NEGATIVE ODOUR NOTICEABLE? | | | | | | |

|  |  |
|---|---|
| 🏠 **COLONY NAME** | |
| 📅 **DATE** | |
| 🕐 **TIME** | |

## WEATHER CONDITIONS

🌡 _____  ☀️  ⛅  🌦  ⛈  ❄️
🚩 _____  ☐  ☐  ☐  ☐  ☐

## INSPECTION

| 🍯 HIVE NUMBER | ① | ② | ③ | ④ | ⑤ | ⑥ |
|---|---|---|---|---|---|---|

## PRODUCTIVITY & REPRODUCTION

| | | | | | | |
|---|---|---|---|---|---|---|
| AMOUNT OF HONEY | | | | | | |
| GENERAL POPULATION | | | | | | |
| AMOUNT OF BROOD | | | | | | |
| AMOUNT OF SPACE | | | | | | |

## BEHAVIOUR & ACTIVITIES

| | | | | | | |
|---|---|---|---|---|---|---|
| USUAL ENTERING AND EXITING ACTIVITY? | | | | | | |
| CALM BEHAVIOUR WHEN OPENING HIVE? | | | | | | |
| BEES BRINGING POLLEN INTO HIVE? | | | | | | |
| SIGNS OF ROBBERY AMONG THE BEES? | | | | | | |

## HEALTH STATUS

| | | | | | | |
|---|---|---|---|---|---|---|
| BEES SEEM WEAK OR LAZY? | | | | | | |
| HIGH AMOUNT OF DEAD BEES? | | | | | | |
| QUEEN BEE IS PRESENT / IDENTIFIABLE? | | | | | | |
| INFESTATION BY ANTS / ANTS PRESENT? | | | | | | |
| INFESTATION BY WAX MOTH / WAX MOTH PRESENT? | | | | | | |
| NEGATIVE ODOUR NOTICEABLE? | | | | | | |

| COLONY NAME | |
|---|---|
| DATE | |
| TIME | |

**WEATHER CONDITIONS**

🌡 ____   ☀  ⛅  🌧  ⛈  ❄
🚩 ____   ☐  ☐  ☐  ☐  ☐

## INSPECTION

| HIVE NUMBER | ① | ② | ③ | ④ | ⑤ | ⑥ |
|---|---|---|---|---|---|---|

## PRODUCTIVITY & REPRODUCTION

| | | | | | | |
|---|---|---|---|---|---|---|
| AMOUNT OF HONEY | | | | | | |
| GENERAL POPULATION | | | | | | |
| AMOUNT OF BROOD | | | | | | |
| AMOUNT OF SPACE | | | | | | |

## BEHAVIOUR & ACTIVITIES

| | | | | | | |
|---|---|---|---|---|---|---|
| USUAL ENTERING AND EXITING ACTIVITY? | | | | | | |
| CALM BEHAVIOUR WHEN OPENING HIVE? | | | | | | |
| BEES BRINGING POLLEN INTO HIVE? | | | | | | |
| SIGNS OF ROBBERY AMONG THE BEES? | | | | | | |

## HEALTH STATUS

| | | | | | | |
|---|---|---|---|---|---|---|
| BEES SEEM WEAK OR LAZY? | | | | | | |
| HIGH AMOUNT OF DEAD BEES? | | | | | | |
| QUEEN BEE IS PRESENT / IDENTIFIABLE? | | | | | | |
| INFESTATION BY ANTS / ANTS PRESENT? | | | | | | |
| INFESTATION BY WAX MOTH / WAX MOTH PRESENT? | | | | | | |
| NEGATIVE ODOUR NOTICEABLE? | | | | | | |

| COLONY NAME | |
|---|---|
| DATE | |
| TIME | |

| WEATHER CONDITIONS | | | | | | |
|---|---|---|---|---|---|---|
| 🌡 ___ | ☀ | ⛅ | 🌧 | ⛈ | ❄ |
| 🚩 ___ | ☐ | ☐ | ☐ | ☐ | ☐ |

## INSPECTION

| HIVE NUMBER | 1 | 2 | 3 | 4 | 5 | 6 |
|---|---|---|---|---|---|---|

## PRODUCTIVITY & REPRODUCTION

| | | | | | | |
|---|---|---|---|---|---|---|
| AMOUNT OF HONEY | | | | | | |
| GENERAL POPULATION | | | | | | |
| AMOUNT OF BROOD | | | | | | |
| AMOUNT OF SPACE | | | | | | |

## BEHAVIOUR & ACTIVITIES

| | | | | | | |
|---|---|---|---|---|---|---|
| USUAL ENTERING AND EXITING ACTIVITY? | | | | | | |
| CALM BEHAVIOUR WHEN OPENING HIVE? | | | | | | |
| BEES BRINGING POLLEN INTO HIVE? | | | | | | |
| SIGNS OF ROBBERY AMONG THE BEES? | | | | | | |

## HEALTH STATUS

| | | | | | | |
|---|---|---|---|---|---|---|
| BEES SEEM WEAK OR LAZY? | | | | | | |
| HIGH AMOUNT OF DEAD BEES? | | | | | | |
| QUEEN BEE IS PRESENT / IDENTIFIABLE? | | | | | | |
| INFESTATION BY ANTS / ANTS PRESENT? | | | | | | |
| INFESTATION BY WAX MOTH / WAX MOTH PRESENT? | | | | | | |
| NEGATIVE ODOUR NOTICEABLE? | | | | | | |

| COLONY NAME | | WEATHER CONDITIONS | | | | | |
|---|---|---|---|---|---|---|---|
| DATE | | 🌡 ____ | ☀ | ⛅ | 🌧 | ⛈ | ❄ |
| TIME | | 🚩 ____ | ☐ | ☐ | ☐ | ☐ | ☐ |

## INSPECTION

| HIVE NUMBER | 1 | 2 | 3 | 4 | 5 | 6 |
|---|---|---|---|---|---|---|

## PRODUCTIVITY & REPRODUCTION

| | | | | | | |
|---|---|---|---|---|---|---|
| AMOUNT OF HONEY | | | | | | |
| GENERAL POPULATION | | | | | | |
| AMOUNT OF BROOD | | | | | | |
| AMOUNT OF SPACE | | | | | | |

## BEHAVIOUR & ACTIVITIES

| | | | | | | |
|---|---|---|---|---|---|---|
| USUAL ENTERING AND EXITING ACTIVITY? | | | | | | |
| CALM BEHAVIOUR WHEN OPENING HIVE? | | | | | | |
| BEES BRINGING POLLEN INTO HIVE? | | | | | | |
| SIGNS OF ROBBERY AMONG THE BEES? | | | | | | |

## HEALTH STATUS

| | | | | | | |
|---|---|---|---|---|---|---|
| BEES SEEM WEAK OR LAZY? | | | | | | |
| HIGH AMOUNT OF DEAD BEES? | | | | | | |
| QUEEN BEE IS PRESENT / IDENTIFIABLE? | | | | | | |
| INFESTATION BY ANTS / ANTS PRESENT? | | | | | | |
| INFESTATION BY WAX MOTH / WAX MOTH PRESENT? | | | | | | |
| NEGATIVE ODOUR NOTICEABLE? | | | | | | |

|  | COLONY NAME |
|---|---|
|  | DATE |
|  | TIME |

**WEATHER CONDITIONS**

🌡 ____  ☀ ☁ 🌧 ⛈ ❄
🚩 ____  ☐ ☐ ☐ ☐ ☐

## INSPECTION

| HIVE NUMBER | ① | ② | ③ | ④ | ⑤ | ⑥ |
|---|---|---|---|---|---|---|

## PRODUCTIVITY & REPRODUCTION

| | | | | | | |
|---|---|---|---|---|---|---|
| AMOUNT OF HONEY | | | | | | |
| GENERAL POPULATION | | | | | | |
| AMOUNT OF BROOD | | | | | | |
| AMOUNT OF SPACE | | | | | | |

## BEHAVIOUR & ACTIVITIES

| | | | | | | |
|---|---|---|---|---|---|---|
| USUAL ENTERING AND EXITING ACTIVITY? | | | | | | |
| CALM BEHAVIOUR WHEN OPENING HIVE? | | | | | | |
| BEES BRINGING POLLEN INTO HIVE? | | | | | | |
| SIGNS OF ROBBERY AMONG THE BEES? | | | | | | |

## HEALTH STATUS

| | | | | | | |
|---|---|---|---|---|---|---|
| BEES SEEM WEAK OR LAZY? | | | | | | |
| HIGH AMOUNT OF DEAD BEES? | | | | | | |
| QUEEN BEE IS PRESENT / IDENTIFIABLE? | | | | | | |
| INFESTATION BY ANTS / ANTS PRESENT? | | | | | | |
| INFESTATION BY WAX MOTH / WAX MOTH PRESENT? | | | | | | |
| NEGATIVE ODOUR NOTICEABLE? | | | | | | |

| COLONY NAME | | WEATHER CONDITIONS | |
|---|---|---|---|
| DATE | | 🌡 ____ ☀ ⛅ 🌧 ⛈ ❄ | |
| TIME | | 🚩 ____ ☐ ☐ ☐ ☐ ☐ | |

## INSPECTION

| HIVE NUMBER | 1 | 2 | 3 | 4 | 5 | 6 |
|---|---|---|---|---|---|---|

## PRODUCTIVITY & REPRODUCTION

| | 1 | 2 | 3 | 4 | 5 | 6 |
|---|---|---|---|---|---|---|
| AMOUNT OF HONEY | | | | | | |
| GENERAL POPULATION | | | | | | |
| AMOUNT OF BROOD | | | | | | |
| AMOUNT OF SPACE | | | | | | |

## BEHAVIOUR & ACTIVITIES

| | 1 | 2 | 3 | 4 | 5 | 6 |
|---|---|---|---|---|---|---|
| USUAL ENTERING AND EXITING ACTIVITY? | | | | | | |
| CALM BEHAVIOUR WHEN OPENING HIVE? | | | | | | |
| BEES BRINGING POLLEN INTO HIVE? | | | | | | |
| SIGNS OF ROBBERY AMONG THE BEES? | | | | | | |

## HEALTH STATUS

| | 1 | 2 | 3 | 4 | 5 | 6 |
|---|---|---|---|---|---|---|
| BEES SEEM WEAK OR LAZY? | | | | | | |
| HIGH AMOUNT OF DEAD BEES? | | | | | | |
| QUEEN BEE IS PRESENT / IDENTIFIABLE? | | | | | | |
| INFESTATION BY ANTS / ANTS PRESENT? | | | | | | |
| INFESTATION BY WAX MOTH / WAX MOTH PRESENT? | | | | | | |
| NEGATIVE ODOUR NOTICEABLE? | | | | | | |

| COLONY NAME | |
|---|---|
| DATE | |
| TIME | |

**WEATHER CONDITIONS**

🌡 _____   ☀ ⛅ 🌧 ⛈ ❄
🏳 _____   ☐ ☐ ☐ ☐ ☐

## INSPECTION

| HIVE NUMBER | ① | ② | ③ | ④ | ⑤ | ⑥ |
|---|---|---|---|---|---|---|

## PRODUCTIVITY & REPRODUCTION

| | | | | | | |
|---|---|---|---|---|---|---|
| AMOUNT OF HONEY | | | | | | |
| GENERAL POPULATION | | | | | | |
| AMOUNT OF BROOD | | | | | | |
| AMOUNT OF SPACE | | | | | | |

## BEHAVIOUR & ACTIVITIES

| | | | | | | |
|---|---|---|---|---|---|---|
| USUAL ENTERING AND EXITING ACTIVITY? | | | | | | |
| CALM BEHAVIOUR WHEN OPENING HIVE? | | | | | | |
| BEES BRINGING POLLEN INTO HIVE? | | | | | | |
| SIGNS OF ROBBERY AMONG THE BEES? | | | | | | |

## HEALTH STATUS

| | | | | | | |
|---|---|---|---|---|---|---|
| BEES SEEM WEAK OR LAZY? | | | | | | |
| HIGH AMOUNT OF DEAD BEES? | | | | | | |
| QUEEN BEE IS PRESENT / IDENTIFIABLE? | | | | | | |
| INFESTATION BY ANTS / ANTS PRESENT? | | | | | | |
| INFESTATION BY WAX MOTH / WAX MOTH PRESENT? | | | | | | |
| NEGATIVE ODOUR NOTICEABLE? | | | | | | |

| | COLONY NAME | | | WEATHER CONDITIONS | | | | |
|---|---|---|---|---|---|---|---|---|
| | DATE | | | ☀ | ⛅ | 🌧 | ⛈ | ❄ |
| | TIME | | | ☐ | ☐ | ☐ | ☐ | ☐ |

## INSPECTION

| HIVE NUMBER | 1 | 2 | 3 | 4 | 5 | 6 |
|---|---|---|---|---|---|---|

### PRODUCTIVITY & REPRODUCTION

| | | | | | | |
|---|---|---|---|---|---|---|
| AMOUNT OF HONEY | | | | | | |
| GENERAL POPULATION | | | | | | |
| AMOUNT OF BROOD | | | | | | |
| AMOUNT OF SPACE | | | | | | |

### BEHAVIOUR & ACTIVITIES

| | | | | | | |
|---|---|---|---|---|---|---|
| USUAL ENTERING AND EXITING ACTIVITY? | | | | | | |
| CALM BEHAVIOUR WHEN OPENING HIVE? | | | | | | |
| BEES BRINGING POLLEN INTO HIVE? | | | | | | |
| SIGNS OF ROBBERY AMONG THE BEES? | | | | | | |

### HEALTH STATUS

| | | | | | | |
|---|---|---|---|---|---|---|
| BEES SEEM WEAK OR LAZY? | | | | | | |
| HIGH AMOUNT OF DEAD BEES? | | | | | | |
| QUEEN BEE IS PRESENT / IDENTIFIABLE? | | | | | | |
| INFESTATION BY ANTS / ANTS PRESENT? | | | | | | |
| INFESTATION BY WAX MOTH / WAX MOTH PRESENT? | | | | | | |
| NEGATIVE ODOUR NOTICEABLE? | | | | | | |

|  |  |
|---|---|
| 🏠 **COLONY NAME** | |
| 📅 **DATE** | |
| 🕐 **TIME** | |

**WEATHER CONDITIONS**

🌡 _____ ☀️ ⛅ 🌧 ⛈ ❄️
🚩 _____ ☐ ☐ ☐ ☐ ☐

## INSPECTION

| HIVE NUMBER | ① | ② | ③ | ④ | ⑤ | ⑥ |
|---|---|---|---|---|---|---|

## PRODUCTIVITY & REPRODUCTION

| | | | | | | |
|---|---|---|---|---|---|---|
| AMOUNT OF HONEY | | | | | | |
| GENERAL POPULATION | | | | | | |
| AMOUNT OF BROOD | | | | | | |
| AMOUNT OF SPACE | | | | | | |

## BEHAVIOUR & ACTIVITIES

| | | | | | | |
|---|---|---|---|---|---|---|
| USUAL ENTERING AND EXITING ACTIVITY? | | | | | | |
| CALM BEHAVIOUR WHEN OPENING HIVE? | | | | | | |
| BEES BRINGING POLLEN INTO HIVE? | | | | | | |
| SIGNS OF ROBBERY AMONG THE BEES? | | | | | | |

## HEALTH STATUS

| | | | | | | |
|---|---|---|---|---|---|---|
| BEES SEEM WEAK OR LAZY? | | | | | | |
| HIGH AMOUNT OF DEAD BEES? | | | | | | |
| QUEEN BEE IS PRESENT / IDENTIFIABLE? | | | | | | |
| INFESTATION BY ANTS / ANTS PRESENT? | | | | | | |
| INFESTATION BY WAX MOTH / WAX MOTH PRESENT? | | | | | | |
| NEGATIVE ODOUR NOTICEABLE? | | | | | | |

|  | COLONY NAME |
|---|---|
|  | DATE |
|  | TIME |

### WEATHER CONDITIONS

| 🌡 | ___ | ☀ | ⛅ | 🌧 | ⛈ | ❄ |
|---|---|---|---|---|---|---|
| 🚩 | ___ | ☐ | ☐ | ☐ | ☐ | ☐ |

### INSPECTION

| HIVE NUMBER | 1 | 2 | 3 | 4 | 5 | 6 |
|---|---|---|---|---|---|---|

### PRODUCTIVITY & REPRODUCTION

| | | | | | | |
|---|---|---|---|---|---|---|
| AMOUNT OF HONEY | | | | | | |
| GENERAL POPULATION | | | | | | |
| AMOUNT OF BROOD | | | | | | |
| AMOUNT OF SPACE | | | | | | |

### BEHAVIOUR & ACTIVITIES

| | | | | | | |
|---|---|---|---|---|---|---|
| USUAL ENTERING AND EXITING ACTIVITY? | | | | | | |
| CALM BEHAVIOUR WHEN OPENING HIVE? | | | | | | |
| BEES BRINGING POLLEN INTO HIVE? | | | | | | |
| SIGNS OF ROBBERY AMONG THE BEES? | | | | | | |

### HEALTH STATUS

| | | | | | | |
|---|---|---|---|---|---|---|
| BEES SEEM WEAK OR LAZY? | | | | | | |
| HIGH AMOUNT OF DEAD BEES? | | | | | | |
| QUEEN BEE IS PRESENT / IDENTIFIABLE? | | | | | | |
| INFESTATION BY ANTS / ANTS PRESENT? | | | | | | |
| INFESTATION BY WAX MOTH / WAX MOTH PRESENT? | | | | | | |
| NEGATIVE ODOUR NOTICEABLE? | | | | | | |

| COLONY NAME | |
|---|---|
| DATE | |
| TIME | |

| WEATHER CONDITIONS | | | | | | |
|---|---|---|---|---|---|---|
| 🌡 ___ | ☀ | ⛅ | 🌧 | ⛈ | ❄ | |
| 🚩 ___ | ☐ | ☐ | ☐ | ☐ | ☐ | |

## INSPECTION

| HIVE NUMBER | 1 | 2 | 3 | 4 | 5 | 6 |
|---|---|---|---|---|---|---|

## PRODUCTIVITY & REPRODUCTION

| | 1 | 2 | 3 | 4 | 5 | 6 |
|---|---|---|---|---|---|---|
| AMOUNT OF HONEY | | | | | | |
| GENERAL POPULATION | | | | | | |
| AMOUNT OF BROOD | | | | | | |
| AMOUNT OF SPACE | | | | | | |

## BEHAVIOUR & ACTIVITIES

| | 1 | 2 | 3 | 4 | 5 | 6 |
|---|---|---|---|---|---|---|
| USUAL ENTERING AND EXITING ACTIVITY? | | | | | | |
| CALM BEHAVIOUR WHEN OPENING HIVE? | | | | | | |
| BEES BRINGING POLLEN INTO HIVE? | | | | | | |
| SIGNS OF ROBBERY AMONG THE BEES? | | | | | | |

## HEALTH STATUS

| | 1 | 2 | 3 | 4 | 5 | 6 |
|---|---|---|---|---|---|---|
| BEES SEEM WEAK OR LAZY? | | | | | | |
| HIGH AMOUNT OF DEAD BEES? | | | | | | |
| QUEEN BEE IS PRESENT / IDENTIFIABLE? | | | | | | |
| INFESTATION BY ANTS / ANTS PRESENT? | | | | | | |
| INFESTATION BY WAX MOTH / WAX MOTH PRESENT? | | | | | | |
| NEGATIVE ODOUR NOTICEABLE? | | | | | | |

|  | COLONY NAME |
|---|---|
|  | DATE |
|  | TIME |

## WEATHER CONDITIONS

🌡 _____ ☀️ ⛅ 🌧 ⛈ ❄️

🪁 _____ ☐ ☐ ☐ ☐ ☐

## INSPECTION

| HIVE NUMBER | ① | ② | ③ | ④ | ⑤ | ⑥ |
|---|---|---|---|---|---|---|

## PRODUCTIVITY & REPRODUCTION

| | | | | | | |
|---|---|---|---|---|---|---|
| AMOUNT OF HONEY | | | | | | |
| GENERAL POPULATION | | | | | | |
| AMOUNT OF BROOD | | | | | | |
| AMOUNT OF SPACE | | | | | | |

## BEHAVIOUR & ACTIVITIES

| | | | | | | |
|---|---|---|---|---|---|---|
| USUAL ENTERING AND EXITING ACTIVITY? | | | | | | |
| CALM BEHAVIOUR WHEN OPENING HIVE? | | | | | | |
| BEES BRINGING POLLEN INTO HIVE? | | | | | | |
| SIGNS OF ROBBERY AMONG THE BEES? | | | | | | |

## HEALTH STATUS

| | | | | | | |
|---|---|---|---|---|---|---|
| BEES SEEM WEAK OR LAZY? | | | | | | |
| HIGH AMOUNT OF DEAD BEES? | | | | | | |
| QUEEN BEE IS PRESENT / IDENTIFIABLE? | | | | | | |
| INFESTATION BY ANTS / ANTS PRESENT? | | | | | | |
| INFESTATION BY WAX MOTH / WAX MOTH PRESENT? | | | | | | |
| NEGATIVE ODOUR NOTICEABLE? | | | | | | |

|  | COLONY NAME |
|---|---|
|  | DATE |
|  | TIME |

## WEATHER CONDITIONS

🌡 ____ ☀ ⛅ 🌧 ⛈ ❄
🚩 ____ ☐ ☐ ☐ ☐ ☐

## INSPECTION

| HIVE NUMBER | 1 | 2 | 3 | 4 | 5 | 6 |
|---|---|---|---|---|---|---|

## PRODUCTIVITY & REPRODUCTION

| | | | | | | |
|---|---|---|---|---|---|---|
| AMOUNT OF HONEY | | | | | | |
| GENERAL POPULATION | | | | | | |
| AMOUNT OF BROOD | | | | | | |
| AMOUNT OF SPACE | | | | | | |

## BEHAVIOUR & ACTIVITIES

| | | | | | | |
|---|---|---|---|---|---|---|
| USUAL ENTERING AND EXITING ACTIVITY? | | | | | | |
| CALM BEHAVIOUR WHEN OPENING HIVE? | | | | | | |
| BEES BRINGING POLLEN INTO HIVE? | | | | | | |
| SIGNS OF ROBBERY AMONG THE BEES? | | | | | | |

## HEALTH STATUS

| | | | | | | |
|---|---|---|---|---|---|---|
| BEES SEEM WEAK OR LAZY? | | | | | | |
| HIGH AMOUNT OF DEAD BEES? | | | | | | |
| QUEEN BEE IS PRESENT / IDENTIFIABLE? | | | | | | |
| INFESTATION BY ANTS / ANTS PRESENT? | | | | | | |
| INFESTATION BY WAX MOTH / WAX MOTH PRESENT? | | | | | | |
| NEGATIVE ODOUR NOTICEABLE? | | | | | | |

|  | COLONY NAME |
|---|---|
|  | DATE |
|  | TIME |

### WEATHER CONDITIONS

| 🌡 | ___ | ☀ ☐ | ⛅ ☐ | 🌧 ☐ | ⛈ ☐ | ❄ ☐ |
|---|---|---|---|---|---|---|
| 🚩 | ___ | | | | | |

### INSPECTION

| HIVE NUMBER | 1 | 2 | 3 | 4 | 5 | 6 |
|---|---|---|---|---|---|---|

### PRODUCTIVITY & REPRODUCTION

| | | | | | | |
|---|---|---|---|---|---|---|
| AMOUNT OF HONEY | | | | | | |
| GENERAL POPULATION | | | | | | |
| AMOUNT OF BROOD | | | | | | |
| AMOUNT OF SPACE | | | | | | |

### BEHAVIOUR & ACTIVITIES

| | | | | | | |
|---|---|---|---|---|---|---|
| USUAL ENTERING AND EXITING ACTIVITY? | | | | | | |
| CALM BEHAVIOUR WHEN OPENING HIVE? | | | | | | |
| BEES BRINGING POLLEN INTO HIVE? | | | | | | |
| SIGNS OF ROBBERY AMONG THE BEES? | | | | | | |

### HEALTH STATUS

| | | | | | | |
|---|---|---|---|---|---|---|
| BEES SEEM WEAK OR LAZY? | | | | | | |
| HIGH AMOUNT OF DEAD BEES? | | | | | | |
| QUEEN BEE IS PRESENT / IDENTIFIABLE? | | | | | | |
| INFESTATION BY ANTS / ANTS PRESENT? | | | | | | |
| INFESTATION BY WAX MOTH / WAX MOTH PRESENT? | | | | | | |
| NEGATIVE ODOUR NOTICEABLE? | | | | | | |

| COLONY NAME | |
|---|---|
| DATE | |
| TIME | |

**WEATHER CONDITIONS**

🌡 _____  ☀ ⛅ 🌧 ⛈ ❄
🚩 _____  ☐ ☐ ☐ ☐ ☐

## INSPECTION

| HIVE NUMBER | ① | ② | ③ | ④ | ⑤ | ⑥ |
|---|---|---|---|---|---|---|

### PRODUCTIVITY & REPRODUCTION

| | | | | | | |
|---|---|---|---|---|---|---|
| AMOUNT OF HONEY | | | | | | |
| GENERAL POPULATION | | | | | | |
| AMOUNT OF BROOD | | | | | | |
| AMOUNT OF SPACE | | | | | | |

### BEHAVIOUR & ACTIVITIES

| | | | | | | |
|---|---|---|---|---|---|---|
| USUAL ENTERING AND EXITING ACTIVITY? | | | | | | |
| CALM BEHAVIOUR WHEN OPENING HIVE? | | | | | | |
| BEES BRINGING POLLEN INTO HIVE? | | | | | | |
| SIGNS OF ROBBERY AMONG THE BEES? | | | | | | |

### HEALTH STATUS

| | | | | | | |
|---|---|---|---|---|---|---|
| BEES SEEM WEAK OR LAZY? | | | | | | |
| HIGH AMOUNT OF DEAD BEES? | | | | | | |
| QUEEN BEE IS PRESENT / IDENTIFIABLE? | | | | | | |
| INFESTATION BY ANTS / ANTS PRESENT? | | | | | | |
| INFESTATION BY WAX MOTH / WAX MOTH PRESENT? | | | | | | |
| NEGATIVE ODOUR NOTICEABLE? | | | | | | |

|  |  |
|---|---|
| 🏠 **COLONY NAME** | |
| 📅 **DATE** | |
| 🕐 **TIME** | |

| **WEATHER CONDITIONS** |
|---|
| 🌡 ____  ☀ ⛅ 🌧 ⛈ ❄ |
| 🚩 ____  ☐ ☐ ☐ ☐ ☐ |

## INSPECTION

| | 1 | 2 | 3 | 4 | 5 | 6 |
|---|---|---|---|---|---|---|
| 🍯 HIVE NUMBER | | | | | | |

## PRODUCTIVITY & REPRODUCTION

| | | | | | | |
|---|---|---|---|---|---|---|
| AMOUNT OF HONEY | | | | | | |
| GENERAL POPULATION | | | | | | |
| AMOUNT OF BROOD | | | | | | |
| AMOUNT OF SPACE | | | | | | |

## BEHAVIOUR & ACTIVITIES

| | | | | | | |
|---|---|---|---|---|---|---|
| USUAL ENTERING AND EXITING ACTIVITY? | | | | | | |
| CALM BEHAVIOUR WHEN OPENING HIVE? | | | | | | |
| BEES BRINGING POLLEN INTO HIVE? | | | | | | |
| SIGNS OF ROBBERY AMONG THE BEES? | | | | | | |

## HEALTH STATUS

| | | | | | | |
|---|---|---|---|---|---|---|
| BEES SEEM WEAK OR LAZY? | | | | | | |
| HIGH AMOUNT OF DEAD BEES? | | | | | | |
| QUEEN BEE IS PRESENT / IDENTIFIABLE? | | | | | | |
| INFESTATION BY ANTS / ANTS PRESENT? | | | | | | |
| INFESTATION BY WAX MOTH / WAX MOTH PRESENT? | | | | | | |
| NEGATIVE ODOUR NOTICEABLE? | | | | | | |

|  | COLONY NAME |
|---|---|
|  | DATE |
|  | TIME |

**WEATHER CONDITIONS**

🌡 ____    ☀️  ⛅  🌧  ⛈  ❄️
🚩 ____    ☐  ☐  ☐  ☐  ☐

## INSPECTION

| HIVE NUMBER | ① | ② | ③ | ④ | ⑤ | ⑥ |
|---|---|---|---|---|---|---|

## PRODUCTIVITY & REPRODUCTION

| | | | | | | |
|---|---|---|---|---|---|---|
| AMOUNT OF HONEY | | | | | | |
| GENERAL POPULATION | | | | | | |
| AMOUNT OF BROOD | | | | | | |
| AMOUNT OF SPACE | | | | | | |

## BEHAVIOUR & ACTIVITIES

| | | | | | | |
|---|---|---|---|---|---|---|
| USUAL ENTERING AND EXITING ACTIVITY? | | | | | | |
| CALM BEHAVIOUR WHEN OPENING HIVE? | | | | | | |
| BEES BRINGING POLLEN INTO HIVE? | | | | | | |
| SIGNS OF ROBBERY AMONG THE BEES? | | | | | | |

## HEALTH STATUS

| | | | | | | |
|---|---|---|---|---|---|---|
| BEES SEEM WEAK OR LAZY? | | | | | | |
| HIGH AMOUNT OF DEAD BEES? | | | | | | |
| QUEEN BEE IS PRESENT / IDENTIFIABLE? | | | | | | |
| INFESTATION BY ANTS / ANTS PRESENT? | | | | | | |
| INFESTATION BY WAX MOTH / WAX MOTH PRESENT? | | | | | | |
| NEGATIVE ODOUR NOTICEABLE? | | | | | | |

| COLONY NAME | | WEATHER CONDITIONS | |
|---|---|---|---|
| DATE | | 🌡 ___ ☀ ⛅ 🌧 ⛈ ❄ | |
| TIME | | 🚩 ___ ☐ ☐ ☐ ☐ ☐ | |

## INSPECTION

| HIVE NUMBER | 1 | 2 | 3 | 4 | 5 | 6 |
|---|---|---|---|---|---|---|

### PRODUCTIVITY & REPRODUCTION

| | 1 | 2 | 3 | 4 | 5 | 6 |
|---|---|---|---|---|---|---|
| AMOUNT OF HONEY | | | | | | |
| GENERAL POPULATION | | | | | | |
| AMOUNT OF BROOD | | | | | | |
| AMOUNT OF SPACE | | | | | | |

### BEHAVIOUR & ACTIVITIES

| | 1 | 2 | 3 | 4 | 5 | 6 |
|---|---|---|---|---|---|---|
| USUAL ENTERING AND EXITING ACTIVITY? | | | | | | |
| CALM BEHAVIOUR WHEN OPENING HIVE? | | | | | | |
| BEES BRINGING POLLEN INTO HIVE? | | | | | | |
| SIGNS OF ROBBERY AMONG THE BEES? | | | | | | |

### HEALTH STATUS

| | 1 | 2 | 3 | 4 | 5 | 6 |
|---|---|---|---|---|---|---|
| BEES SEEM WEAK OR LAZY? | | | | | | |
| HIGH AMOUNT OF DEAD BEES? | | | | | | |
| QUEEN BEE IS PRESENT / IDENTIFIABLE? | | | | | | |
| INFESTATION BY ANTS / ANTS PRESENT? | | | | | | |
| INFESTATION BY WAX MOTH / WAX MOTH PRESENT? | | | | | | |
| NEGATIVE ODOUR NOTICEABLE? | | | | | | |

|  | COLONY NAME |
|---|---|
|  | DATE |
|  | TIME |

**WEATHER CONDITIONS**

🌡 ———   ☀  ⛅  🌧  ⛈  ❄
🚩 ———   ☐  ☐  ☐  ☐  ☐

## INSPECTION

| HIVE NUMBER | ① | ② | ③ | ④ | ⑤ | ⑥ |
|---|---|---|---|---|---|---|

## PRODUCTIVITY & REPRODUCTION

| | | | | | | |
|---|---|---|---|---|---|---|
| AMOUNT OF HONEY | | | | | | |
| GENERAL POPULATION | | | | | | |
| AMOUNT OF BROOD | | | | | | |
| AMOUNT OF SPACE | | | | | | |

## BEHAVIOUR & ACTIVITIES

| | | | | | | |
|---|---|---|---|---|---|---|
| USUAL ENTERING AND EXITING ACTIVITY? | | | | | | |
| CALM BEHAVIOUR WHEN OPENING HIVE? | | | | | | |
| BEES BRINGING POLLEN INTO HIVE? | | | | | | |
| SIGNS OF ROBBERY AMONG THE BEES? | | | | | | |

## HEALTH STATUS

| | | | | | | |
|---|---|---|---|---|---|---|
| BEES SEEM WEAK OR LAZY? | | | | | | |
| HIGH AMOUNT OF DEAD BEES? | | | | | | |
| QUEEN BEE IS PRESENT / IDENTIFIABLE? | | | | | | |
| INFESTATION BY ANTS / ANTS PRESENT? | | | | | | |
| INFESTATION BY WAX MOTH / WAX MOTH PRESENT? | | | | | | |
| NEGATIVE ODOUR NOTICEABLE? | | | | | | |

| COLONY NAME | |
|---|---|
| DATE | |
| TIME | |

**WEATHER CONDITIONS**

🌡️ _____  ☀️  ⛅  🌧️  ⛈️  ❄️

🚩 _____  ☐  ☐  ☐  ☐  ☐

## INSPECTION

| HIVE NUMBER | ① | ② | ③ | ④ | ⑤ | ⑥ |
|---|---|---|---|---|---|---|

## PRODUCTIVITY & REPRODUCTION

| | | | | | | |
|---|---|---|---|---|---|---|
| AMOUNT OF HONEY | | | | | | |
| GENERAL POPULATION | | | | | | |
| AMOUNT OF BROOD | | | | | | |
| AMOUNT OF SPACE | | | | | | |

## BEHAVIOUR & ACTIVITIES

| | | | | | | |
|---|---|---|---|---|---|---|
| USUAL ENTERING AND EXITING ACTIVITY? | | | | | | |
| CALM BEHAVIOUR WHEN OPENING HIVE? | | | | | | |
| BEES BRINGING POLLEN INTO HIVE? | | | | | | |
| SIGNS OF ROBBERY AMONG THE BEES? | | | | | | |

## HEALTH STATUS

| | | | | | | |
|---|---|---|---|---|---|---|
| BEES SEEM WEAK OR LAZY? | | | | | | |
| HIGH AMOUNT OF DEAD BEES? | | | | | | |
| QUEEN BEE IS PRESENT / IDENTIFIABLE? | | | | | | |
| INFESTATION BY ANTS / ANTS PRESENT? | | | | | | |
| INFESTATION BY WAX MOTH / WAX MOTH PRESENT? | | | | | | |
| NEGATIVE ODOUR NOTICEABLE? | | | | | | |

| COLONY NAME | |
|---|---|
| DATE | |
| TIME | |

## WEATHER CONDITIONS

| 🌡 ___ | ☀ | ⛅ | 🌦 | 🌧 | ❄ |
|---|---|---|---|---|---|
| 🚩 ___ | ☐ | ☐ | ☐ | ☐ | ☐ |

## INSPECTION

| HIVE NUMBER | ① | ② | ③ | ④ | ⑤ | ⑥ |
|---|---|---|---|---|---|---|

## PRODUCTIVITY & REPRODUCTION

| | | | | | | |
|---|---|---|---|---|---|---|
| AMOUNT OF HONEY | | | | | | |
| GENERAL POPULATION | | | | | | |
| AMOUNT OF BROOD | | | | | | |
| AMOUNT OF SPACE | | | | | | |

## BEHAVIOUR & ACTIVITIES

| | | | | | | |
|---|---|---|---|---|---|---|
| USUAL ENTERING AND EXITING ACTIVITY? | | | | | | |
| CALM BEHAVIOUR WHEN OPENING HIVE? | | | | | | |
| BEES BRINGING POLLEN INTO HIVE? | | | | | | |
| SIGNS OF ROBBERY AMONG THE BEES? | | | | | | |

## HEALTH STATUS

| | | | | | | |
|---|---|---|---|---|---|---|
| BEES SEEM WEAK OR LAZY? | | | | | | |
| HIGH AMOUNT OF DEAD BEES? | | | | | | |
| QUEEN BEE IS PRESENT / IDENTIFIABLE? | | | | | | |
| INFESTATION BY ANTS / ANTS PRESENT? | | | | | | |
| INFESTATION BY WAX MOTH / WAX MOTH PRESENT? | | | | | | |
| NEGATIVE ODOUR NOTICEABLE? | | | | | | |

| | COLONY NAME |
|---|---|
| | DATE |
| | TIME |

## WEATHER CONDITIONS

🌡 _____  ☀ ☁ 🌧 ⛈ ❄
🚩 _____  ☐ ☐ ☐ ☐ ☐

## INSPECTION

| HIVE NUMBER | 1 | 2 | 3 | 4 | 5 | 6 |
|---|---|---|---|---|---|---|

## PRODUCTIVITY & REPRODUCTION

| | | | | | | |
|---|---|---|---|---|---|---|
| AMOUNT OF HONEY | | | | | | |
| GENERAL POPULATION | | | | | | |
| AMOUNT OF BROOD | | | | | | |
| AMOUNT OF SPACE | | | | | | |

## BEHAVIOUR & ACTIVITIES

| | | | | | | |
|---|---|---|---|---|---|---|
| USUAL ENTERING AND EXITING ACTIVITY? | | | | | | |
| CALM BEHAVIOUR WHEN OPENING HIVE? | | | | | | |
| BEES BRINGING POLLEN INTO HIVE? | | | | | | |
| SIGNS OF ROBBERY AMONG THE BEES? | | | | | | |

## HEALTH STATUS

| | | | | | | |
|---|---|---|---|---|---|---|
| BEES SEEM WEAK OR LAZY? | | | | | | |
| HIGH AMOUNT OF DEAD BEES? | | | | | | |
| QUEEN BEE IS PRESENT / IDENTIFIABLE? | | | | | | |
| INFESTATION BY ANTS / ANTS PRESENT? | | | | | | |
| INFESTATION BY WAX MOTH / WAX MOTH PRESENT? | | | | | | |
| NEGATIVE ODOUR NOTICEABLE? | | | | | | |

| COLONY NAME | |
|---|---|
| DATE | |
| TIME | |

**WEATHER CONDITIONS**

🌡 ____    ☀ ☁ 🌧 ⛈ ❄
🚩 ____    ☐ ☐ ☐ ☐ ☐

## INSPECTION

| HIVE NUMBER | ① | ② | ③ | ④ | ⑤ | ⑥ |
|---|---|---|---|---|---|---|

## PRODUCTIVITY & REPRODUCTION

| | | | | | | |
|---|---|---|---|---|---|---|
| AMOUNT OF HONEY | | | | | | |
| GENERAL POPULATION | | | | | | |
| AMOUNT OF BROOD | | | | | | |
| AMOUNT OF SPACE | | | | | | |

## BEHAVIOUR & ACTIVITIES

| | | | | | | |
|---|---|---|---|---|---|---|
| USUAL ENTERING AND EXITING ACTIVITY? | | | | | | |
| CALM BEHAVIOUR WHEN OPENING HIVE? | | | | | | |
| BEES BRINGING POLLEN INTO HIVE? | | | | | | |
| SIGNS OF ROBBERY AMONG THE BEES? | | | | | | |

## HEALTH STATUS

| | | | | | | |
|---|---|---|---|---|---|---|
| BEES SEEM WEAK OR LAZY? | | | | | | |
| HIGH AMOUNT OF DEAD BEES? | | | | | | |
| QUEEN BEE IS PRESENT / IDENTIFIABLE? | | | | | | |
| INFESTATION BY ANTS / ANTS PRESENT? | | | | | | |
| INFESTATION BY WAX MOTH / WAX MOTH PRESENT? | | | | | | |
| NEGATIVE ODOUR NOTICEABLE? | | | | | | |

| COLONY NAME | |
|---|---|
| DATE | |
| TIME | |

## WEATHER CONDITIONS

🌡 _____  ☀ ☁ 🌧 ⛈ ❄
🚩 _____  ☐ ☐ ☐ ☐ ☐

## INSPECTION

| HIVE NUMBER | 1 | 2 | 3 | 4 | 5 | 6 |
|---|---|---|---|---|---|---|

## PRODUCTIVITY & REPRODUCTION

| | | | | | | |
|---|---|---|---|---|---|---|
| AMOUNT OF HONEY | | | | | | |
| GENERAL POPULATION | | | | | | |
| AMOUNT OF BROOD | | | | | | |
| AMOUNT OF SPACE | | | | | | |

## BEHAVIOUR & ACTIVITIES

| | | | | | | |
|---|---|---|---|---|---|---|
| USUAL ENTERING AND EXITING ACTIVITY? | | | | | | |
| CALM BEHAVIOUR WHEN OPENING HIVE? | | | | | | |
| BEES BRINGING POLLEN INTO HIVE? | | | | | | |
| SIGNS OF ROBBERY AMONG THE BEES? | | | | | | |

## HEALTH STATUS

| | | | | | | |
|---|---|---|---|---|---|---|
| BEES SEEM WEAK OR LAZY? | | | | | | |
| HIGH AMOUNT OF DEAD BEES? | | | | | | |
| QUEEN BEE IS PRESENT / IDENTIFIABLE? | | | | | | |
| INFESTATION BY ANTS / ANTS PRESENT? | | | | | | |
| INFESTATION BY WAX MOTH / WAX MOTH PRESENT? | | | | | | |
| NEGATIVE ODOUR NOTICEABLE? | | | | | | |

| COLONY NAME | |
|---|---|
| DATE | |
| TIME | |

**WEATHER CONDITIONS**

🌡 _____  ☀  ⛅  🌧  ⛈  ❄
🚩 _____  ☐  ☐  ☐  ☐  ☐

## INSPECTION

| HIVE NUMBER | ① | ② | ③ | ④ | ⑤ | ⑥ |
|---|---|---|---|---|---|---|

## PRODUCTIVITY & REPRODUCTION

| | | | | | | |
|---|---|---|---|---|---|---|
| AMOUNT OF HONEY | | | | | | |
| GENERAL POPULATION | | | | | | |
| AMOUNT OF BROOD | | | | | | |
| AMOUNT OF SPACE | | | | | | |

## BEHAVIOUR & ACTIVITIES

| | | | | | | |
|---|---|---|---|---|---|---|
| USUAL ENTERING AND EXITING ACTIVITY? | | | | | | |
| CALM BEHAVIOUR WHEN OPENING HIVE? | | | | | | |
| BEES BRINGING POLLEN INTO HIVE? | | | | | | |
| SIGNS OF ROBBERY AMONG THE BEES? | | | | | | |

## HEALTH STATUS

| | | | | | | |
|---|---|---|---|---|---|---|
| BEES SEEM WEAK OR LAZY? | | | | | | |
| HIGH AMOUNT OF DEAD BEES? | | | | | | |
| QUEEN BEE IS PRESENT / IDENTIFIABLE? | | | | | | |
| INFESTATION BY ANTS / ANTS PRESENT? | | | | | | |
| INFESTATION BY WAX MOTH / WAX MOTH PRESENT? | | | | | | |
| NEGATIVE ODOUR NOTICEABLE? | | | | | | |

|  | COLONY NAME |
|---|---|
|  | DATE |
|  | TIME |

### WEATHER CONDITIONS

| 🌡 | ___ | ☀ | ⛅ | 🌧 | ⛈ | ❄ |
|---|---|---|---|---|---|---|
| 🚩 | ___ | ☐ | ☐ | ☐ | ☐ | ☐ |

### INSPECTION

| HIVE NUMBER | ① | ② | ③ | ④ | ⑤ | ⑥ |
|---|---|---|---|---|---|---|

### PRODUCTIVITY & REPRODUCTION

| | | | | | | |
|---|---|---|---|---|---|---|
| AMOUNT OF HONEY | | | | | | |
| GENERAL POPULATION | | | | | | |
| AMOUNT OF BROOD | | | | | | |
| AMOUNT OF SPACE | | | | | | |

### BEHAVIOUR & ACTIVITIES

| | | | | | | |
|---|---|---|---|---|---|---|
| USUAL ENTERING AND EXITING ACTIVITY? | | | | | | |
| CALM BEHAVIOUR WHEN OPENING HIVE? | | | | | | |
| BEES BRINGING POLLEN INTO HIVE? | | | | | | |
| SIGNS OF ROBBERY AMONG THE BEES? | | | | | | |

### HEALTH STATUS

| | | | | | | |
|---|---|---|---|---|---|---|
| BEES SEEM WEAK OR LAZY? | | | | | | |
| HIGH AMOUNT OF DEAD BEES? | | | | | | |
| QUEEN BEE IS PRESENT / IDENTIFIABLE? | | | | | | |
| INFESTATION BY ANTS / ANTS PRESENT? | | | | | | |
| INFESTATION BY WAX MOTH / WAX MOTH PRESENT? | | | | | | |
| NEGATIVE ODOUR NOTICEABLE? | | | | | | |

|  | COLONY NAME |
|---|---|
|  | DATE |
|  | TIME |

## WEATHER CONDITIONS

🌡 _____   ☀  ⛅  🌧  ⛈  ❄
🚩 _____   ☐  ☐  ☐  ☐  ☐

## INSPECTION

| HIVE NUMBER | ① | ② | ③ | ④ | ⑤ | ⑥ |
|---|---|---|---|---|---|---|

### PRODUCTIVITY & REPRODUCTION

| | | | | | | |
|---|---|---|---|---|---|---|
| AMOUNT OF HONEY | | | | | | |
| GENERAL POPULATION | | | | | | |
| AMOUNT OF BROOD | | | | | | |
| AMOUNT OF SPACE | | | | | | |

### BEHAVIOUR & ACTIVITIES

| | | | | | | |
|---|---|---|---|---|---|---|
| USUAL ENTERING AND EXITING ACTIVITY? | | | | | | |
| CALM BEHAVIOUR WHEN OPENING HIVE? | | | | | | |
| BEES BRINGING POLLEN INTO HIVE? | | | | | | |
| SIGNS OF ROBBERY AMONG THE BEES? | | | | | | |

### HEALTH STATUS

| | | | | | | |
|---|---|---|---|---|---|---|
| BEES SEEM WEAK OR LAZY? | | | | | | |
| HIGH AMOUNT OF DEAD BEES? | | | | | | |
| QUEEN BEE IS PRESENT / IDENTIFIABLE? | | | | | | |
| INFESTATION BY ANTS / ANTS PRESENT? | | | | | | |
| INFESTATION BY WAX MOTH / WAX MOTH PRESENT? | | | | | | |
| NEGATIVE ODOUR NOTICEABLE? | | | | | | |

| COLONY NAME | |
|---|---|
| DATE | |
| TIME | |

**WEATHER CONDITIONS**

🌡 ____ ☀ ⛅ ☁ ⛈ ❄
🚩 ____ ☐ ☐ ☐ ☐ ☐

## INSPECTION

| HIVE NUMBER | 1 | 2 | 3 | 4 | 5 | 6 |
|---|---|---|---|---|---|---|

## PRODUCTIVITY & REPRODUCTION

| | | | | | | |
|---|---|---|---|---|---|---|
| AMOUNT OF HONEY | | | | | | |
| GENERAL POPULATION | | | | | | |
| AMOUNT OF BROOD | | | | | | |
| AMOUNT OF SPACE | | | | | | |

## BEHAVIOUR & ACTIVITIES

| | | | | | | |
|---|---|---|---|---|---|---|
| USUAL ENTERING AND EXITING ACTIVITY? | | | | | | |
| CALM BEHAVIOUR WHEN OPENING HIVE? | | | | | | |
| BEES BRINGING POLLEN INTO HIVE? | | | | | | |
| SIGNS OF ROBBERY AMONG THE BEES? | | | | | | |

## HEALTH STATUS

| | | | | | | |
|---|---|---|---|---|---|---|
| BEES SEEM WEAK OR LAZY? | | | | | | |
| HIGH AMOUNT OF DEAD BEES? | | | | | | |
| QUEEN BEE IS PRESENT / IDENTIFIABLE? | | | | | | |
| INFESTATION BY ANTS / ANTS PRESENT? | | | | | | |
| INFESTATION BY WAX MOTH / WAX MOTH PRESENT? | | | | | | |
| NEGATIVE ODOUR NOTICEABLE? | | | | | | |

| COLONY NAME | |
|---|---|
| DATE | |
| TIME | |

**WEATHER CONDITIONS**

🌡 ____ ☀ ⛅ 🌧 ⛈ ❄
🚩 ____ ☐ ☐ ☐ ☐ ☐

## INSPECTION

| HIVE NUMBER | ① | ② | ③ | ④ | ⑤ | ⑥ |
|---|---|---|---|---|---|---|

## PRODUCTIVITY & REPRODUCTION

| | | | | | | |
|---|---|---|---|---|---|---|
| AMOUNT OF HONEY | | | | | | |
| GENERAL POPULATION | | | | | | |
| AMOUNT OF BROOD | | | | | | |
| AMOUNT OF SPACE | | | | | | |

## BEHAVIOUR & ACTIVITIES

| | | | | | | |
|---|---|---|---|---|---|---|
| USUAL ENTERING AND EXITING ACTIVITY? | | | | | | |
| CALM BEHAVIOUR WHEN OPENING HIVE? | | | | | | |
| BEES BRINGING POLLEN INTO HIVE? | | | | | | |
| SIGNS OF ROBBERY AMONG THE BEES? | | | | | | |

## HEALTH STATUS

| | | | | | | |
|---|---|---|---|---|---|---|
| BEES SEEM WEAK OR LAZY? | | | | | | |
| HIGH AMOUNT OF DEAD BEES? | | | | | | |
| QUEEN BEE IS PRESENT / IDENTIFIABLE? | | | | | | |
| INFESTATION BY ANTS / ANTS PRESENT? | | | | | | |
| INFESTATION BY WAX MOTH / WAX MOTH PRESENT? | | | | | | |
| NEGATIVE ODOUR NOTICEABLE? | | | | | | |

| COLONY NAME | |
|---|---|
| DATE | |
| TIME | |

**WEATHER CONDITIONS**

🌡 ____   ☀ ⛅ 🌧 ⛈ ❄
🚩 ____   ☐ ☐ ☐ ☐ ☐

## INSPECTION

| HIVE NUMBER | ① | ② | ③ | ④ | ⑤ | ⑥ |
|---|---|---|---|---|---|---|

## PRODUCTIVITY & REPRODUCTION

| | | | | | | |
|---|---|---|---|---|---|---|
| AMOUNT OF HONEY | | | | | | |
| GENERAL POPULATION | | | | | | |
| AMOUNT OF BROOD | | | | | | |
| AMOUNT OF SPACE | | | | | | |

## BEHAVIOUR & ACTIVITIES

| | | | | | | |
|---|---|---|---|---|---|---|
| USUAL ENTERING AND EXITING ACTIVITY? | | | | | | |
| CALM BEHAVIOUR WHEN OPENING HIVE? | | | | | | |
| BEES BRINGING POLLEN INTO HIVE? | | | | | | |
| SIGNS OF ROBBERY AMONG THE BEES? | | | | | | |

## HEALTH STATUS

| | | | | | | |
|---|---|---|---|---|---|---|
| BEES SEEM WEAK OR LAZY? | | | | | | |
| HIGH AMOUNT OF DEAD BEES? | | | | | | |
| QUEEN BEE IS PRESENT / IDENTIFIABLE? | | | | | | |
| INFESTATION BY ANTS / ANTS PRESENT? | | | | | | |
| INFESTATION BY WAX MOTH / WAX MOTH PRESENT? | | | | | | |
| NEGATIVE ODOUR NOTICEABLE? | | | | | | |

| | COLONY NAME |
|---|---|
| | DATE |
| | TIME |

**WEATHER CONDITIONS**

🌡 _____   ☀ ☁ 🌧 ⛈ ❄
🚩 _____   ☐ ☐ ☐ ☐ ☐

## INSPECTION

| HIVE NUMBER | ① | ② | ③ | ④ | ⑤ | ⑥ |
|---|---|---|---|---|---|---|

## PRODUCTIVITY & REPRODUCTION

| | | | | | | |
|---|---|---|---|---|---|---|
| AMOUNT OF HONEY | | | | | | |
| GENERAL POPULATION | | | | | | |
| AMOUNT OF BROOD | | | | | | |
| AMOUNT OF SPACE | | | | | | |

## BEHAVIOUR & ACTIVITIES

| | | | | | | |
|---|---|---|---|---|---|---|
| USUAL ENTERING AND EXITING ACTIVITY? | | | | | | |
| CALM BEHAVIOUR WHEN OPENING HIVE? | | | | | | |
| BEES BRINGING POLLEN INTO HIVE? | | | | | | |
| SIGNS OF ROBBERY AMONG THE BEES? | | | | | | |

## HEALTH STATUS

| | | | | | | |
|---|---|---|---|---|---|---|
| BEES SEEM WEAK OR LAZY? | | | | | | |
| HIGH AMOUNT OF DEAD BEES? | | | | | | |
| QUEEN BEE IS PRESENT / IDENTIFIABLE? | | | | | | |
| INFESTATION BY ANTS / ANTS PRESENT? | | | | | | |
| INFESTATION BY WAX MOTH / WAX MOTH PRESENT? | | | | | | |
| NEGATIVE ODOUR NOTICEABLE? | | | | | | |

| COLONY NAME | |
|---|---|
| DATE | |
| TIME | |

## WEATHER CONDITIONS

🌡 _____  ☀ ☁ 🌧 ⛈ ❄
🚩 _____  ☐ ☐ ☐ ☐

## INSPECTION

| HIVE NUMBER | ① | ② | ③ | ④ | ⑤ | ⑥ |
|---|---|---|---|---|---|---|

## PRODUCTIVITY & REPRODUCTION

| | | | | | | |
|---|---|---|---|---|---|---|
| AMOUNT OF HONEY | | | | | | |
| GENERAL POPULATION | | | | | | |
| AMOUNT OF BROOD | | | | | | |
| AMOUNT OF SPACE | | | | | | |

## BEHAVIOUR & ACTIVITIES

| | | | | | | |
|---|---|---|---|---|---|---|
| USUAL ENTERING AND EXITING ACTIVITY? | | | | | | |
| CALM BEHAVIOUR WHEN OPENING HIVE? | | | | | | |
| BEES BRINGING POLLEN INTO HIVE? | | | | | | |
| SIGNS OF ROBBERY AMONG THE BEES? | | | | | | |

## HEALTH STATUS

| | | | | | | |
|---|---|---|---|---|---|---|
| BEES SEEM WEAK OR LAZY? | | | | | | |
| HIGH AMOUNT OF DEAD BEES? | | | | | | |
| QUEEN BEE IS PRESENT / IDENTIFIABLE? | | | | | | |
| INFESTATION BY ANTS / ANTS PRESENT? | | | | | | |
| INFESTATION BY WAX MOTH / WAX MOTH PRESENT? | | | | | | |
| NEGATIVE ODOUR NOTICEABLE? | | | | | | |

| COLONY NAME | |
|---|---|
| DATE | |
| TIME | |

**WEATHER CONDITIONS**

🌡 ____   ☀ ☁ 🌧 ⛈ ❄
🚩 ____   ☐ ☐ ☐ ☐ ☐

## INSPECTION

| HIVE NUMBER | ① | ② | ③ | ④ | ⑤ | ⑥ |
|---|---|---|---|---|---|---|

## PRODUCTIVITY & REPRODUCTION

| | | | | | | |
|---|---|---|---|---|---|---|
| AMOUNT OF HONEY | | | | | | |
| GENERAL POPULATION | | | | | | |
| AMOUNT OF BROOD | | | | | | |
| AMOUNT OF SPACE | | | | | | |

## BEHAVIOUR & ACTIVITIES

| | | | | | | |
|---|---|---|---|---|---|---|
| USUAL ENTERING AND EXITING ACTIVITY? | | | | | | |
| CALM BEHAVIOUR WHEN OPENING HIVE? | | | | | | |
| BEES BRINGING POLLEN INTO HIVE? | | | | | | |
| SIGNS OF ROBBERY AMONG THE BEES? | | | | | | |

## HEALTH STATUS

| | | | | | | |
|---|---|---|---|---|---|---|
| BEES SEEM WEAK OR LAZY? | | | | | | |
| HIGH AMOUNT OF DEAD BEES? | | | | | | |
| QUEEN BEE IS PRESENT / IDENTIFIABLE? | | | | | | |
| INFESTATION BY ANTS / ANTS PRESENT? | | | | | | |
| INFESTATION BY WAX MOTH / WAX MOTH PRESENT? | | | | | | |
| NEGATIVE ODOUR NOTICEABLE? | | | | | | |

| COLONY NAME | |
|---|---|
| DATE | |
| TIME | |

| WEATHER CONDITIONS | | | | | | |
|---|---|---|---|---|---|---|
| 🌡 ___ | | ☀ | ⛅ | 🌧 | ⛈ | ❄ |
| 🚩 ___ | | ☐ | ☐ | ☐ | ☐ | ☐ |

## INSPECTION

| HIVE NUMBER | ① | ② | ③ | ④ | ⑤ | ⑥ |
|---|---|---|---|---|---|---|

## PRODUCTIVITY & REPRODUCTION

| | 1 | 2 | 3 | 4 | 5 | 6 |
|---|---|---|---|---|---|---|
| AMOUNT OF HONEY | | | | | | |
| GENERAL POPULATION | | | | | | |
| AMOUNT OF BROOD | | | | | | |
| AMOUNT OF SPACE | | | | | | |

## BEHAVIOUR & ACTIVITIES

| | 1 | 2 | 3 | 4 | 5 | 6 |
|---|---|---|---|---|---|---|
| USUAL ENTERING AND EXITING ACTIVITY? | | | | | | |
| CALM BEHAVIOUR WHEN OPENING HIVE? | | | | | | |
| BEES BRINGING POLLEN INTO HIVE? | | | | | | |
| SIGNS OF ROBBERY AMONG THE BEES? | | | | | | |

## HEALTH STATUS

| | 1 | 2 | 3 | 4 | 5 | 6 |
|---|---|---|---|---|---|---|
| BEES SEEM WEAK OR LAZY? | | | | | | |
| HIGH AMOUNT OF DEAD BEES? | | | | | | |
| QUEEN BEE IS PRESENT / IDENTIFIABLE? | | | | | | |
| INFESTATION BY ANTS / ANTS PRESENT? | | | | | | |
| INFESTATION BY WAX MOTH / WAX MOTH PRESENT? | | | | | | |
| NEGATIVE ODOUR NOTICEABLE? | | | | | | |

|  | COLONY NAME |
|---|---|
|  | DATE |
|  | TIME |

**WEATHER CONDITIONS**

🌡 ——   ☀  ⛅  🌦  ⛈  ❄
🚩 ——   ☐  ☐  ☐  ☐  ☐

## INSPECTION

| HIVE NUMBER | ① | ② | ③ | ④ | ⑤ | ⑥ |
|---|---|---|---|---|---|---|

## PRODUCTIVITY & REPRODUCTION

| | | | | | | |
|---|---|---|---|---|---|---|
| AMOUNT OF HONEY | | | | | | |
| GENERAL POPULATION | | | | | | |
| AMOUNT OF BROOD | | | | | | |
| AMOUNT OF SPACE | | | | | | |

## BEHAVIOUR & ACTIVITIES

| | | | | | | |
|---|---|---|---|---|---|---|
| USUAL ENTERING AND EXITING ACTIVITY? | | | | | | |
| CALM BEHAVIOUR WHEN OPENING HIVE? | | | | | | |
| BEES BRINGING POLLEN INTO HIVE? | | | | | | |
| SIGNS OF ROBBERY AMONG THE BEES? | | | | | | |

## HEALTH STATUS

| | | | | | | |
|---|---|---|---|---|---|---|
| BEES SEEM WEAK OR LAZY? | | | | | | |
| HIGH AMOUNT OF DEAD BEES? | | | | | | |
| QUEEN BEE IS PRESENT / IDENTIFIABLE? | | | | | | |
| INFESTATION BY ANTS / ANTS PRESENT? | | | | | | |
| INFESTATION BY WAX MOTH / WAX MOTH PRESENT? | | | | | | |
| NEGATIVE ODOUR NOTICEABLE? | | | | | | |

| COLONY NAME | |
|---|---|
| DATE | |
| TIME | |

**WEATHER CONDITIONS**

🌡 _____  ☀  ⛅  🌧  ⛈  ❄
🚩 _____  ☐  ☐  ☐  ☐  ☐

## INSPECTION

| HIVE NUMBER | ① | ② | ③ | ④ | ⑤ | ⑥ |
|---|---|---|---|---|---|---|

### PRODUCTIVITY & REPRODUCTION

| | | | | | | |
|---|---|---|---|---|---|---|
| AMOUNT OF HONEY | | | | | | |
| GENERAL POPULATION | | | | | | |
| AMOUNT OF BROOD | | | | | | |
| AMOUNT OF SPACE | | | | | | |

### BEHAVIOUR & ACTIVITIES

| | | | | | | |
|---|---|---|---|---|---|---|
| USUAL ENTERING AND EXITING ACTIVITY? | | | | | | |
| CALM BEHAVIOUR WHEN OPENING HIVE? | | | | | | |
| BEES BRINGING POLLEN INTO HIVE? | | | | | | |
| SIGNS OF ROBBERY AMONG THE BEES? | | | | | | |

### HEALTH STATUS

| | | | | | | |
|---|---|---|---|---|---|---|
| BEES SEEM WEAK OR LAZY? | | | | | | |
| HIGH AMOUNT OF DEAD BEES? | | | | | | |
| QUEEN BEE IS PRESENT / IDENTIFIABLE? | | | | | | |
| INFESTATION BY ANTS / ANTS PRESENT? | | | | | | |
| INFESTATION BY WAX MOTH / WAX MOTH PRESENT? | | | | | | |
| NEGATIVE ODOUR NOTICEABLE? | | | | | | |

|  | COLONY NAME |
|---|---|
|  | DATE |
|  | TIME |

### WEATHER CONDITIONS

🌡 _____   ☀  ⛅  🌧  ⛈  ❄
🚩 _____   ☐  ☐  ☐  ☐  ☐

### INSPECTION

| HIVE NUMBER | 1 | 2 | 3 | 4 | 5 | 6 |
|---|---|---|---|---|---|---|

### PRODUCTIVITY & REPRODUCTION

| | | | | | | |
|---|---|---|---|---|---|---|
| AMOUNT OF HONEY | | | | | | |
| GENERAL POPULATION | | | | | | |
| AMOUNT OF BROOD | | | | | | |
| AMOUNT OF SPACE | | | | | | |

### BEHAVIOUR & ACTIVITIES

| | | | | | | |
|---|---|---|---|---|---|---|
| USUAL ENTERING AND EXITING ACTIVITY? | | | | | | |
| CALM BEHAVIOUR WHEN OPENING HIVE? | | | | | | |
| BEES BRINGING POLLEN INTO HIVE? | | | | | | |
| SIGNS OF ROBBERY AMONG THE BEES? | | | | | | |

### HEALTH STATUS

| | | | | | | |
|---|---|---|---|---|---|---|
| BEES SEEM WEAK OR LAZY? | | | | | | |
| HIGH AMOUNT OF DEAD BEES? | | | | | | |
| QUEEN BEE IS PRESENT / IDENTIFIABLE? | | | | | | |
| INFESTATION BY ANTS / ANTS PRESENT? | | | | | | |
| INFESTATION BY WAX MOTH / WAX MOTH PRESENT? | | | | | | |
| NEGATIVE ODOUR NOTICEABLE? | | | | | | |

|  | COLONY NAME |
|---|---|
|  | DATE |
|  | TIME |

**WEATHER CONDITIONS**

🌡 ____  ☀ ⛅ 🌧 ⛈ ❄
🚩 ____  ☐ ☐ ☐ ☐ ☐

## INSPECTION

| HIVE NUMBER | 1 | 2 | 3 | 4 | 5 | 6 |
|---|---|---|---|---|---|---|

## PRODUCTIVITY & REPRODUCTION

| | 1 | 2 | 3 | 4 | 5 | 6 |
|---|---|---|---|---|---|---|
| AMOUNT OF HONEY | | | | | | |
| GENERAL POPULATION | | | | | | |
| AMOUNT OF BROOD | | | | | | |
| AMOUNT OF SPACE | | | | | | |

## BEHAVIOUR & ACTIVITIES

| | 1 | 2 | 3 | 4 | 5 | 6 |
|---|---|---|---|---|---|---|
| USUAL ENTERING AND EXITING ACTIVITY? | | | | | | |
| CALM BEHAVIOUR WHEN OPENING HIVE? | | | | | | |
| BEES BRINGING POLLEN INTO HIVE? | | | | | | |
| SIGNS OF ROBBERY AMONG THE BEES? | | | | | | |

## HEALTH STATUS

| | 1 | 2 | 3 | 4 | 5 | 6 |
|---|---|---|---|---|---|---|
| BEES SEEM WEAK OR LAZY? | | | | | | |
| HIGH AMOUNT OF DEAD BEES? | | | | | | |
| QUEEN BEE IS PRESENT / IDENTIFIABLE? | | | | | | |
| INFESTATION BY ANTS / ANTS PRESENT? | | | | | | |
| INFESTATION BY WAX MOTH / WAX MOTH PRESENT? | | | | | | |
| NEGATIVE ODOUR NOTICEABLE? | | | | | | |

|  | COLONY NAME |
|---|---|
|  | DATE |
|  | TIME |

**WEATHER CONDITIONS**

🌡 _____ ☀ ⛅ 🌧 ⛈ ❄
🚩 _____ ☐ ☐ ☐ ☐ ☐

## INSPECTION

| HIVE NUMBER | ① | ② | ③ | ④ | ⑤ | ⑥ |
|---|---|---|---|---|---|---|

## PRODUCTIVITY & REPRODUCTION

| | | | | | | |
|---|---|---|---|---|---|---|
| AMOUNT OF HONEY | | | | | | |
| GENERAL POPULATION | | | | | | |
| AMOUNT OF BROOD | | | | | | |
| AMOUNT OF SPACE | | | | | | |

## BEHAVIOUR & ACTIVITIES

| | | | | | | |
|---|---|---|---|---|---|---|
| USUAL ENTERING AND EXITING ACTIVITY? | | | | | | |
| CALM BEHAVIOUR WHEN OPENING HIVE? | | | | | | |
| BEES BRINGING POLLEN INTO HIVE? | | | | | | |
| SIGNS OF ROBBERY AMONG THE BEES? | | | | | | |

## HEALTH STATUS

| | | | | | | |
|---|---|---|---|---|---|---|
| BEES SEEM WEAK OR LAZY? | | | | | | |
| HIGH AMOUNT OF DEAD BEES? | | | | | | |
| QUEEN BEE IS PRESENT / IDENTIFIABLE? | | | | | | |
| INFESTATION BY ANTS / ANTS PRESENT? | | | | | | |
| INFESTATION BY WAX MOTH / WAX MOTH PRESENT? | | | | | | |
| NEGATIVE ODOUR NOTICEABLE? | | | | | | |

| COLONY NAME | |
|---|---|
| DATE | |
| TIME | |

## WEATHER CONDITIONS

🌡 ____    ☀ ☁ 🌧 ⛈ ❄
🚩 ____    ☐ ☐ ☐ ☐ ☐

## INSPECTION

| HIVE NUMBER | ① | ② | ③ | ④ | ⑤ | ⑥ |
|---|---|---|---|---|---|---|

## PRODUCTIVITY & REPRODUCTION

| | | | | | | |
|---|---|---|---|---|---|---|
| AMOUNT OF HONEY | | | | | | |
| GENERAL POPULATION | | | | | | |
| AMOUNT OF BROOD | | | | | | |
| AMOUNT OF SPACE | | | | | | |

## BEHAVIOUR & ACTIVITIES

| | | | | | | |
|---|---|---|---|---|---|---|
| USUAL ENTERING AND EXITING ACTIVITY? | | | | | | |
| CALM BEHAVIOUR WHEN OPENING HIVE? | | | | | | |
| BEES BRINGING POLLEN INTO HIVE? | | | | | | |
| SIGNS OF ROBBERY AMONG THE BEES? | | | | | | |

## HEALTH STATUS

| | | | | | | |
|---|---|---|---|---|---|---|
| BEES SEEM WEAK OR LAZY? | | | | | | |
| HIGH AMOUNT OF DEAD BEES? | | | | | | |
| QUEEN BEE IS PRESENT / IDENTIFIABLE? | | | | | | |
| INFESTATION BY ANTS / ANTS PRESENT? | | | | | | |
| INFESTATION BY WAX MOTH / WAX MOTH PRESENT? | | | | | | |
| NEGATIVE ODOUR NOTICEABLE? | | | | | | |

| COLONY NAME | |
|---|---|
| DATE | |
| TIME | |

**WEATHER CONDITIONS**

🌡 ____  ☀ ⛅ 🌧 ⛈ ❄
🚩 ____  ☐ ☐ ☐ ☐ ☐

## INSPECTION

| HIVE NUMBER | ① | ② | ③ | ④ | ⑤ | ⑥ |
|---|---|---|---|---|---|---|

## PRODUCTIVITY & REPRODUCTION

| | | | | | | |
|---|---|---|---|---|---|---|
| AMOUNT OF HONEY | | | | | | |
| GENERAL POPULATION | | | | | | |
| AMOUNT OF BROOD | | | | | | |
| AMOUNT OF SPACE | | | | | | |

## BEHAVIOUR & ACTIVITIES

| | | | | | | |
|---|---|---|---|---|---|---|
| USUAL ENTERING AND EXITING ACTIVITY? | | | | | | |
| CALM BEHAVIOUR WHEN OPENING HIVE? | | | | | | |
| BEES BRINGING POLLEN INTO HIVE? | | | | | | |
| SIGNS OF ROBBERY AMONG THE BEES? | | | | | | |

## HEALTH STATUS

| | | | | | | |
|---|---|---|---|---|---|---|
| BEES SEEM WEAK OR LAZY? | | | | | | |
| HIGH AMOUNT OF DEAD BEES? | | | | | | |
| QUEEN BEE IS PRESENT / IDENTIFIABLE? | | | | | | |
| INFESTATION BY ANTS / ANTS PRESENT? | | | | | | |
| INFESTATION BY WAX MOTH / WAX MOTH PRESENT? | | | | | | |
| NEGATIVE ODOUR NOTICEABLE? | | | | | | |

|  | COLONY NAME |
|---|---|
|  | DATE |
|  | TIME |

**WEATHER CONDITIONS**

🌡 _____  ☀  ⛅  🌧  ⛈  ❄
🚩 _____  ☐  ☐  ☐  ☐  ☐

## INSPECTION

| HIVE NUMBER | ① | ② | ③ | ④ | ⑤ | ⑥ |
|---|---|---|---|---|---|---|

### PRODUCTIVITY & REPRODUCTION

| | | | | | | |
|---|---|---|---|---|---|---|
| AMOUNT OF HONEY | | | | | | |
| GENERAL POPULATION | | | | | | |
| AMOUNT OF BROOD | | | | | | |
| AMOUNT OF SPACE | | | | | | |

### BEHAVIOUR & ACTIVITIES

| | | | | | | |
|---|---|---|---|---|---|---|
| USUAL ENTERING AND EXITING ACTIVITY? | | | | | | |
| CALM BEHAVIOUR WHEN OPENING HIVE? | | | | | | |
| BEES BRINGING POLLEN INTO HIVE? | | | | | | |
| SIGNS OF ROBBERY AMONG THE BEES? | | | | | | |

### HEALTH STATUS

| | | | | | | |
|---|---|---|---|---|---|---|
| BEES SEEM WEAK OR LAZY? | | | | | | |
| HIGH AMOUNT OF DEAD BEES? | | | | | | |
| QUEEN BEE IS PRESENT / IDENTIFIABLE? | | | | | | |
| INFESTATION BY ANTS / ANTS PRESENT? | | | | | | |
| INFESTATION BY WAX MOTH / WAX MOTH PRESENT? | | | | | | |
| NEGATIVE ODOUR NOTICEABLE? | | | | | | |

| COLONY NAME |
|---|
| DATE |
| TIME |

## WEATHER CONDITIONS

🌡 _____   ☀  ⛅  🌧  ⛈  ❄
🚩 _____   ☐  ☐  ☐  ☐  ☐

## INSPECTION

| HIVE NUMBER | ① | ② | ③ | ④ | ⑤ | ⑥ |
|---|---|---|---|---|---|---|

## PRODUCTIVITY & REPRODUCTION

| | | | | | | |
|---|---|---|---|---|---|---|
| AMOUNT OF HONEY | | | | | | |
| GENERAL POPULATION | | | | | | |
| AMOUNT OF BROOD | | | | | | |
| AMOUNT OF SPACE | | | | | | |

## BEHAVIOUR & ACTIVITIES

| | | | | | | |
|---|---|---|---|---|---|---|
| USUAL ENTERING AND EXITING ACTIVITY? | | | | | | |
| CALM BEHAVIOUR WHEN OPENING HIVE? | | | | | | |
| BEES BRINGING POLLEN INTO HIVE? | | | | | | |
| SIGNS OF ROBBERY AMONG THE BEES? | | | | | | |

## HEALTH STATUS

| | | | | | | |
|---|---|---|---|---|---|---|
| BEES SEEM WEAK OR LAZY? | | | | | | |
| HIGH AMOUNT OF DEAD BEES? | | | | | | |
| QUEEN BEE IS PRESENT / IDENTIFIABLE? | | | | | | |
| INFESTATION BY ANTS / ANTS PRESENT? | | | | | | |
| INFESTATION BY WAX MOTH / WAX MOTH PRESENT? | | | | | | |
| NEGATIVE ODOUR NOTICEABLE? | | | | | | |

| COLONY NAME | |
|---|---|
| DATE | |
| TIME | |

### WEATHER CONDITIONS

🌡 ——   ☀️  ⛅  🌧  ⛈  ❄️
🚩 ——   ☐  ☐  ☐  ☐  ☐

## INSPECTION

| HIVE NUMBER | ① | ② | ③ | ④ | ⑤ | ⑥ |
|---|---|---|---|---|---|---|

### PRODUCTIVITY & REPRODUCTION

| | | | | | | |
|---|---|---|---|---|---|---|
| AMOUNT OF HONEY | | | | | | |
| GENERAL POPULATION | | | | | | |
| AMOUNT OF BROOD | | | | | | |
| AMOUNT OF SPACE | | | | | | |

### BEHAVIOUR & ACTIVITIES

| | | | | | | |
|---|---|---|---|---|---|---|
| USUAL ENTERING AND EXITING ACTIVITY? | | | | | | |
| CALM BEHAVIOUR WHEN OPENING HIVE? | | | | | | |
| BEES BRINGING POLLEN INTO HIVE? | | | | | | |
| SIGNS OF ROBBERY AMONG THE BEES? | | | | | | |

### HEALTH STATUS

| | | | | | | |
|---|---|---|---|---|---|---|
| BEES SEEM WEAK OR LAZY? | | | | | | |
| HIGH AMOUNT OF DEAD BEES? | | | | | | |
| QUEEN BEE IS PRESENT / IDENTIFIABLE? | | | | | | |
| INFESTATION BY ANTS / ANTS PRESENT? | | | | | | |
| INFESTATION BY WAX MOTH / WAX MOTH PRESENT? | | | | | | |
| NEGATIVE ODOUR NOTICEABLE? | | | | | | |

| COLONY NAME | | WEATHER CONDITIONS | | | | | |
|---|---|---|---|---|---|---|---|
| DATE | | 🌡 ___ | ☀ | ⛅ | 🌧 | ⛈ | ❄ |
| TIME | | 🚩 ___ | ☐ | ☐ | ☐ | ☐ | ☐ |

## INSPECTION

| HIVE NUMBER | 1 | 2 | 3 | 4 | 5 | 6 |
|---|---|---|---|---|---|---|

## PRODUCTIVITY & REPRODUCTION

| | | | | | | |
|---|---|---|---|---|---|---|
| AMOUNT OF HONEY | | | | | | |
| GENERAL POPULATION | | | | | | |
| AMOUNT OF BROOD | | | | | | |
| AMOUNT OF SPACE | | | | | | |

## BEHAVIOUR & ACTIVITIES

| | | | | | | |
|---|---|---|---|---|---|---|
| USUAL ENTERING AND EXITING ACTIVITY? | | | | | | |
| CALM BEHAVIOUR WHEN OPENING HIVE? | | | | | | |
| BEES BRINGING POLLEN INTO HIVE? | | | | | | |
| SIGNS OF ROBBERY AMONG THE BEES? | | | | | | |

## HEALTH STATUS

| | | | | | | |
|---|---|---|---|---|---|---|
| BEES SEEM WEAK OR LAZY? | | | | | | |
| HIGH AMOUNT OF DEAD BEES? | | | | | | |
| QUEEN BEE IS PRESENT / IDENTIFIABLE? | | | | | | |
| INFESTATION BY ANTS / ANTS PRESENT? | | | | | | |
| INFESTATION BY WAX MOTH / WAX MOTH PRESENT? | | | | | | |
| NEGATIVE ODOUR NOTICEABLE? | | | | | | |

| COLONY NAME | | WEATHER CONDITIONS | |
|---|---|---|---|
| DATE | | 🌡 ___ | ☀ ⛅ 🌧 ⛈ ❄ |
| TIME | | 🚩 ___ | ☐ ☐ ☐ ☐ ☐ |

## INSPECTION

| | 1 | 2 | 3 | 4 | 5 | 6 |
|---|---|---|---|---|---|---|
| HIVE NUMBER | | | | | | |

## PRODUCTIVITY & REPRODUCTION

| | | | | | | |
|---|---|---|---|---|---|---|
| AMOUNT OF HONEY | | | | | | |
| GENERAL POPULATION | | | | | | |
| AMOUNT OF BROOD | | | | | | |
| AMOUNT OF SPACE | | | | | | |

## BEHAVIOUR & ACTIVITIES

| | | | | | | |
|---|---|---|---|---|---|---|
| USUAL ENTERING AND EXITING ACTIVITY? | | | | | | |
| CALM BEHAVIOUR WHEN OPENING HIVE? | | | | | | |
| BEES BRINGING POLLEN INTO HIVE? | | | | | | |
| SIGNS OF ROBBERY AMONG THE BEES? | | | | | | |

## HEALTH STATUS

| | | | | | | |
|---|---|---|---|---|---|---|
| BEES SEEM WEAK OR LAZY? | | | | | | |
| HIGH AMOUNT OF DEAD BEES? | | | | | | |
| QUEEN BEE IS PRESENT / IDENTIFIABLE? | | | | | | |
| INFESTATION BY ANTS / ANTS PRESENT? | | | | | | |
| INFESTATION BY WAX MOTH / WAX MOTH PRESENT? | | | | | | |
| NEGATIVE ODOUR NOTICEABLE? | | | | | | |

| COLONY NAME | |
|---|---|
| DATE | |
| TIME | |

## WEATHER CONDITIONS

🌡 _____ ☀ ⛅ 🌧 ⛈ ❄
🚩 _____ ☐ ☐ ☐ ☐ ☐

## INSPECTION

| HIVE NUMBER | ① | ② | ③ | ④ | ⑤ | ⑥ |
|---|---|---|---|---|---|---|

## PRODUCTIVITY & REPRODUCTION

| | | | | | | |
|---|---|---|---|---|---|---|
| AMOUNT OF HONEY | | | | | | |
| GENERAL POPULATION | | | | | | |
| AMOUNT OF BROOD | | | | | | |
| AMOUNT OF SPACE | | | | | | |

## BEHAVIOUR & ACTIVITIES

| | | | | | | |
|---|---|---|---|---|---|---|
| USUAL ENTERING AND EXITING ACTIVITY? | | | | | | |
| CALM BEHAVIOUR WHEN OPENING HIVE? | | | | | | |
| BEES BRINGING POLLEN INTO HIVE? | | | | | | |
| SIGNS OF ROBBERY AMONG THE BEES? | | | | | | |

## HEALTH STATUS

| | | | | | | |
|---|---|---|---|---|---|---|
| BEES SEEM WEAK OR LAZY? | | | | | | |
| HIGH AMOUNT OF DEAD BEES? | | | | | | |
| QUEEN BEE IS PRESENT / IDENTIFIABLE? | | | | | | |
| INFESTATION BY ANTS / ANTS PRESENT? | | | | | | |
| INFESTATION BY WAX MOTH / WAX MOTH PRESENT? | | | | | | |
| NEGATIVE ODOUR NOTICEABLE? | | | | | | |

|  | COLONY NAME |
|---|---|
|  | DATE |
|  | TIME |

**WEATHER CONDITIONS**

🌡 _____  ☀ ☁ 🌧 ⛈ ❄
🚩 _____  ☐ ☐ ☐ ☐ ☐

## INSPECTION

| HIVE NUMBER | 1 | 2 | 3 | 4 | 5 | 6 |
|---|---|---|---|---|---|---|

## PRODUCTIVITY & REPRODUCTION

| | | | | | | |
|---|---|---|---|---|---|---|
| AMOUNT OF HONEY | | | | | | |
| GENERAL POPULATION | | | | | | |
| AMOUNT OF BROOD | | | | | | |
| AMOUNT OF SPACE | | | | | | |

## BEHAVIOUR & ACTIVITIES

| | | | | | | |
|---|---|---|---|---|---|---|
| USUAL ENTERING AND EXITING ACTIVITY? | | | | | | |
| CALM BEHAVIOUR WHEN OPENING HIVE? | | | | | | |
| BEES BRINGING POLLEN INTO HIVE? | | | | | | |
| SIGNS OF ROBBERY AMONG THE BEES? | | | | | | |

## HEALTH STATUS

| | | | | | | |
|---|---|---|---|---|---|---|
| BEES SEEM WEAK OR LAZY? | | | | | | |
| HIGH AMOUNT OF DEAD BEES? | | | | | | |
| QUEEN BEE IS PRESENT / IDENTIFIABLE? | | | | | | |
| INFESTATION BY ANTS / ANTS PRESENT? | | | | | | |
| INFESTATION BY WAX MOTH / WAX MOTH PRESENT? | | | | | | |
| NEGATIVE ODOUR NOTICEABLE? | | | | | | |

|  | COLONY NAME |
|---|---|
|  | DATE |
|  | TIME |

## WEATHER CONDITIONS

🌡 _____   ☀️ ⛅ 🌧 ⛈ ❄️
🚩 _____   ☐ ☐ ☐ ☐ ☐

## INSPECTION

| HIVE NUMBER | ① | ② | ③ | ④ | ⑤ | ⑥ |
|---|---|---|---|---|---|---|

## PRODUCTIVITY & REPRODUCTION

| | | | | | | |
|---|---|---|---|---|---|---|
| AMOUNT OF HONEY | | | | | | |
| GENERAL POPULATION | | | | | | |
| AMOUNT OF BROOD | | | | | | |
| AMOUNT OF SPACE | | | | | | |

## BEHAVIOUR & ACTIVITIES

| | | | | | | |
|---|---|---|---|---|---|---|
| USUAL ENTERING AND EXITING ACTIVITY? | | | | | | |
| CALM BEHAVIOUR WHEN OPENING HIVE? | | | | | | |
| BEES BRINGING POLLEN INTO HIVE? | | | | | | |
| SIGNS OF ROBBERY AMONG THE BEES? | | | | | | |

## HEALTH STATUS

| | | | | | | |
|---|---|---|---|---|---|---|
| BEES SEEM WEAK OR LAZY? | | | | | | |
| HIGH AMOUNT OF DEAD BEES? | | | | | | |
| QUEEN BEE IS PRESENT / IDENTIFIABLE? | | | | | | |
| INFESTATION BY ANTS / ANTS PRESENT? | | | | | | |
| INFESTATION BY WAX MOTH / WAX MOTH PRESENT? | | | | | | |
| NEGATIVE ODOUR NOTICEABLE? | | | | | | |

| COLONY NAME | |
|---|---|
| DATE | |
| TIME | |

## WEATHER CONDITIONS

🌡 _____  ☀  ⛅  🌧  ⛈  ❄
🚩 _____  ☐  ☐  ☐  ☐  ☐

## INSPECTION

| HIVE NUMBER | ① | ② | ③ | ④ | ⑤ | ⑥ |
|---|---|---|---|---|---|---|

## PRODUCTIVITY & REPRODUCTION

| | | | | | | |
|---|---|---|---|---|---|---|
| AMOUNT OF HONEY | | | | | | |
| GENERAL POPULATION | | | | | | |
| AMOUNT OF BROOD | | | | | | |
| AMOUNT OF SPACE | | | | | | |

## BEHAVIOUR & ACTIVITIES

| | | | | | | |
|---|---|---|---|---|---|---|
| USUAL ENTERING AND EXITING ACTIVITY? | | | | | | |
| CALM BEHAVIOUR WHEN OPENING HIVE? | | | | | | |
| BEES BRINGING POLLEN INTO HIVE? | | | | | | |
| SIGNS OF ROBBERY AMONG THE BEES? | | | | | | |

## HEALTH STATUS

| | | | | | | |
|---|---|---|---|---|---|---|
| BEES SEEM WEAK OR LAZY? | | | | | | |
| HIGH AMOUNT OF DEAD BEES? | | | | | | |
| QUEEN BEE IS PRESENT / IDENTIFIABLE? | | | | | | |
| INFESTATION BY ANTS / ANTS PRESENT? | | | | | | |
| INFESTATION BY WAX MOTH / WAX MOTH PRESENT? | | | | | | |
| NEGATIVE ODOUR NOTICEABLE? | | | | | | |

| | COLONY NAME |
|---|---|
| | DATE |
| | TIME |

## WEATHER CONDITIONS

🌡 _____  ☀ ⛅ 🌧 ⛈ ❄
🚩 _____  ☐ ☐ ☐ ☐ ☐

## INSPECTION

| HIVE NUMBER | ① | ② | ③ | ④ | ⑤ | ⑥ |
|---|---|---|---|---|---|---|

## PRODUCTIVITY & REPRODUCTION

| | | | | | | |
|---|---|---|---|---|---|---|
| AMOUNT OF HONEY | | | | | | |
| GENERAL POPULATION | | | | | | |
| AMOUNT OF BROOD | | | | | | |
| AMOUNT OF SPACE | | | | | | |

## BEHAVIOUR & ACTIVITIES

| | | | | | | |
|---|---|---|---|---|---|---|
| USUAL ENTERING AND EXITING ACTIVITY? | | | | | | |
| CALM BEHAVIOUR WHEN OPENING HIVE? | | | | | | |
| BEES BRINGING POLLEN INTO HIVE? | | | | | | |
| SIGNS OF ROBBERY AMONG THE BEES? | | | | | | |

## HEALTH STATUS

| | | | | | | |
|---|---|---|---|---|---|---|
| BEES SEEM WEAK OR LAZY? | | | | | | |
| HIGH AMOUNT OF DEAD BEES? | | | | | | |
| QUEEN BEE IS PRESENT / IDENTIFIABLE? | | | | | | |
| INFESTATION BY ANTS / ANTS PRESENT? | | | | | | |
| INFESTATION BY WAX MOTH / WAX MOTH PRESENT? | | | | | | |
| NEGATIVE ODOUR NOTICEABLE? | | | | | | |

|  | COLONY NAME |
|---|---|
|  | DATE |
|  | TIME |

**WEATHER CONDITIONS**

🌡 ____ ☀ ⛅ 🌧 ⛈ ❄
🚩 ____ ☐ ☐ ☐ ☐ ☐

## INSPECTION

| HIVE NUMBER | 1 | 2 | 3 | 4 | 5 | 6 |
|---|---|---|---|---|---|---|

## PRODUCTIVITY & REPRODUCTION

| | 1 | 2 | 3 | 4 | 5 | 6 |
|---|---|---|---|---|---|---|
| AMOUNT OF HONEY | | | | | | |
| GENERAL POPULATION | | | | | | |
| AMOUNT OF BROOD | | | | | | |
| AMOUNT OF SPACE | | | | | | |

## BEHAVIOUR & ACTIVITIES

| | 1 | 2 | 3 | 4 | 5 | 6 |
|---|---|---|---|---|---|---|
| USUAL ENTERING AND EXITING ACTIVITY? | | | | | | |
| CALM BEHAVIOUR WHEN OPENING HIVE? | | | | | | |
| BEES BRINGING POLLEN INTO HIVE? | | | | | | |
| SIGNS OF ROBBERY AMONG THE BEES? | | | | | | |

## HEALTH STATUS

| | 1 | 2 | 3 | 4 | 5 | 6 |
|---|---|---|---|---|---|---|
| BEES SEEM WEAK OR LAZY? | | | | | | |
| HIGH AMOUNT OF DEAD BEES? | | | | | | |
| QUEEN BEE IS PRESENT / IDENTIFIABLE? | | | | | | |
| INFESTATION BY ANTS / ANTS PRESENT? | | | | | | |
| INFESTATION BY WAX MOTH / WAX MOTH PRESENT? | | | | | | |
| NEGATIVE ODOUR NOTICEABLE? | | | | | | |

|  | COLONY NAME |
|---|---|
|  | DATE |
|  | TIME |

**WEATHER CONDITIONS**

🌡 _____  ☀️ ⛅ 🌧 ⛈ ❄️
🚩 _____  ☐ ☐ ☐ ☐ ☐

## INSPECTION

| HIVE NUMBER | ① | ② | ③ | ④ | ⑤ | ⑥ |
|---|---|---|---|---|---|---|

## PRODUCTIVITY & REPRODUCTION

| | | | | | | |
|---|---|---|---|---|---|---|
| AMOUNT OF HONEY | | | | | | |
| GENERAL POPULATION | | | | | | |
| AMOUNT OF BROOD | | | | | | |
| AMOUNT OF SPACE | | | | | | |

## BEHAVIOUR & ACTIVITIES

| | | | | | | |
|---|---|---|---|---|---|---|
| USUAL ENTERING AND EXITING ACTIVITY? | | | | | | |
| CALM BEHAVIOUR WHEN OPENING HIVE? | | | | | | |
| BEES BRINGING POLLEN INTO HIVE? | | | | | | |
| SIGNS OF ROBBERY AMONG THE BEES? | | | | | | |

## HEALTH STATUS

| | | | | | | |
|---|---|---|---|---|---|---|
| BEES SEEM WEAK OR LAZY? | | | | | | |
| HIGH AMOUNT OF DEAD BEES? | | | | | | |
| QUEEN BEE IS PRESENT / IDENTIFIABLE? | | | | | | |
| INFESTATION BY ANTS / ANTS PRESENT? | | | | | | |
| INFESTATION BY WAX MOTH / WAX MOTH PRESENT? | | | | | | |
| NEGATIVE ODOUR NOTICEABLE? | | | | | | |

|  | COLONY NAME |
|---|---|
|  | DATE |
|  | TIME |

## WEATHER CONDITIONS

🌡 _____  ☀  ⛅  🌧  ⛈  ❄
🚩 _____  ☐  ☐  ☐  ☐  ☐

### INSPECTION

| HIVE NUMBER | ① | ② | ③ | ④ | ⑤ | ⑥ |
|---|---|---|---|---|---|---|

### PRODUCTIVITY & REPRODUCTION

| | | | | | | |
|---|---|---|---|---|---|---|
| AMOUNT OF HONEY | | | | | | |
| GENERAL POPULATION | | | | | | |
| AMOUNT OF BROOD | | | | | | |
| AMOUNT OF SPACE | | | | | | |

### BEHAVIOUR & ACTIVITIES

| | | | | | | |
|---|---|---|---|---|---|---|
| USUAL ENTERING AND EXITING ACTIVITY? | | | | | | |
| CALM BEHAVIOUR WHEN OPENING HIVE? | | | | | | |
| BEES BRINGING POLLEN INTO HIVE? | | | | | | |
| SIGNS OF ROBBERY AMONG THE BEES? | | | | | | |

### HEALTH STATUS

| | | | | | | |
|---|---|---|---|---|---|---|
| BEES SEEM WEAK OR LAZY? | | | | | | |
| HIGH AMOUNT OF DEAD BEES? | | | | | | |
| QUEEN BEE IS PRESENT / IDENTIFIABLE? | | | | | | |
| INFESTATION BY ANTS / ANTS PRESENT? | | | | | | |
| INFESTATION BY WAX MOTH / WAX MOTH PRESENT? | | | | | | |
| NEGATIVE ODOUR NOTICEABLE? | | | | | | |

|  | COLONY NAME |
|---|---|
|  | DATE |
|  | TIME |

**WEATHER CONDITIONS**

| 🌡 ___ | ☀ | ⛅ | 🌦 | ⛈ | ❄ |
|---|---|---|---|---|---|
| 🚩 ___ | ☐ | ☐ | ☐ | ☐ | ☐ |

## INSPECTION

| HIVE NUMBER | 1 | 2 | 3 | 4 | 5 | 6 |
|---|---|---|---|---|---|---|

### PRODUCTIVITY & REPRODUCTION

| | | | | | | |
|---|---|---|---|---|---|---|
| AMOUNT OF HONEY | | | | | | |
| GENERAL POPULATION | | | | | | |
| AMOUNT OF BROOD | | | | | | |
| AMOUNT OF SPACE | | | | | | |

### BEHAVIOUR & ACTIVITIES

| | | | | | | |
|---|---|---|---|---|---|---|
| USUAL ENTERING AND EXITING ACTIVITY? | | | | | | |
| CALM BEHAVIOUR WHEN OPENING HIVE? | | | | | | |
| BEES BRINGING POLLEN INTO HIVE? | | | | | | |
| SIGNS OF ROBBERY AMONG THE BEES? | | | | | | |

### HEALTH STATUS

| | | | | | | |
|---|---|---|---|---|---|---|
| BEES SEEM WEAK OR LAZY? | | | | | | |
| HIGH AMOUNT OF DEAD BEES? | | | | | | |
| QUEEN BEE IS PRESENT / IDENTIFIABLE? | | | | | | |
| INFESTATION BY ANTS / ANTS PRESENT? | | | | | | |
| INFESTATION BY WAX MOTH / WAX MOTH PRESENT? | | | | | | |
| NEGATIVE ODOUR NOTICEABLE? | | | | | | |

| COLONY NAME | |
|---|---|
| DATE | |
| TIME | |

| WEATHER CONDITIONS | | | | | | |
|---|---|---|---|---|---|---|
| 🌡 ___ | | ☀ | ⛅ | 🌧 | ⛈ | ❄ |
| 🚩 ___ | | ☐ | ☐ | ☐ | ☐ | ☐ |

## INSPECTION

| HIVE NUMBER | 1 | 2 | 3 | 4 | 5 | 6 |
|---|---|---|---|---|---|---|

### PRODUCTIVITY & REPRODUCTION

| | | | | | | |
|---|---|---|---|---|---|---|
| AMOUNT OF HONEY | | | | | | |
| GENERAL POPULATION | | | | | | |
| AMOUNT OF BROOD | | | | | | |
| AMOUNT OF SPACE | | | | | | |

### BEHAVIOUR & ACTIVITIES

| | | | | | | |
|---|---|---|---|---|---|---|
| USUAL ENTERING AND EXITING ACTIVITY? | | | | | | |
| CALM BEHAVIOUR WHEN OPENING HIVE? | | | | | | |
| BEES BRINGING POLLEN INTO HIVE? | | | | | | |
| SIGNS OF ROBBERY AMONG THE BEES? | | | | | | |

### HEALTH STATUS

| | | | | | | |
|---|---|---|---|---|---|---|
| BEES SEEM WEAK OR LAZY? | | | | | | |
| HIGH AMOUNT OF DEAD BEES? | | | | | | |
| QUEEN BEE IS PRESENT / IDENTIFIABLE? | | | | | | |
| INFESTATION BY ANTS / ANTS PRESENT? | | | | | | |
| INFESTATION BY WAX MOTH / WAX MOTH PRESENT? | | | | | | |
| NEGATIVE ODOUR NOTICEABLE? | | | | | | |

| COLONY NAME | | WEATHER CONDITIONS | | | | | |
|---|---|---|---|---|---|---|---|
| DATE | | 🌡 ___ | ☀ | ⛅ | 🌧 | ⛈ | ❄ |
| TIME | | 🚩 ___ | ☐ | ☐ | ☐ | ☐ | ☐ |

## INSPECTION

| HIVE NUMBER | 1 | 2 | 3 | 4 | 5 | 6 |
|---|---|---|---|---|---|---|

## PRODUCTIVITY & REPRODUCTION

| | | | | | | |
|---|---|---|---|---|---|---|
| AMOUNT OF HONEY | | | | | | |
| GENERAL POPULATION | | | | | | |
| AMOUNT OF BROOD | | | | | | |
| AMOUNT OF SPACE | | | | | | |

## BEHAVIOUR & ACTIVITIES

| | | | | | | |
|---|---|---|---|---|---|---|
| USUAL ENTERING AND EXITING ACTIVITY? | | | | | | |
| CALM BEHAVIOUR WHEN OPENING HIVE? | | | | | | |
| BEES BRINGING POLLEN INTO HIVE? | | | | | | |
| SIGNS OF ROBBERY AMONG THE BEES? | | | | | | |

## HEALTH STATUS

| | | | | | | |
|---|---|---|---|---|---|---|
| BEES SEEM WEAK OR LAZY? | | | | | | |
| HIGH AMOUNT OF DEAD BEES? | | | | | | |
| QUEEN BEE IS PRESENT / IDENTIFIABLE? | | | | | | |
| INFESTATION BY ANTS / ANTS PRESENT? | | | | | | |
| INFESTATION BY WAX MOTH / WAX MOTH PRESENT? | | | | | | |
| NEGATIVE ODOUR NOTICEABLE? | | | | | | |

| COLONY NAME | | WEATHER CONDITIONS | | | | | |
|---|---|---|---|---|---|---|---|
| DATE | | 🌡 ___ | ☀ | ⛅ | 🌧 | ⛈ | ❄ |
| TIME | | 🚩 ___ | ☐ | ☐ | ☐ | ☐ | ☐ |

## INSPECTION

| HIVE NUMBER | 1 | 2 | 3 | 4 | 5 | 6 |
|---|---|---|---|---|---|---|

## PRODUCTIVITY & REPRODUCTION

| | | | | | | |
|---|---|---|---|---|---|---|
| AMOUNT OF HONEY | | | | | | |
| GENERAL POPULATION | | | | | | |
| AMOUNT OF BROOD | | | | | | |
| AMOUNT OF SPACE | | | | | | |

## BEHAVIOUR & ACTIVITIES

| | | | | | | |
|---|---|---|---|---|---|---|
| USUAL ENTERING AND EXITING ACTIVITY? | | | | | | |
| CALM BEHAVIOUR WHEN OPENING HIVE? | | | | | | |
| BEES BRINGING POLLEN INTO HIVE? | | | | | | |
| SIGNS OF ROBBERY AMONG THE BEES? | | | | | | |

## HEALTH STATUS

| | | | | | | |
|---|---|---|---|---|---|---|
| BEES SEEM WEAK OR LAZY? | | | | | | |
| HIGH AMOUNT OF DEAD BEES? | | | | | | |
| QUEEN BEE IS PRESENT / IDENTIFIABLE? | | | | | | |
| INFESTATION BY ANTS / ANTS PRESENT? | | | | | | |
| INFESTATION BY WAX MOTH / WAX MOTH PRESENT? | | | | | | |
| NEGATIVE ODOUR NOTICEABLE? | | | | | | |

|  | COLONY NAME |
|---|---|
|  | DATE |
|  | TIME |

### WEATHER CONDITIONS

| 🌡 | ___ | ☀ | ⛅ | 🌧 | ⛈ | ❄ |
|---|---|---|---|---|---|---|
| 🚩 | ___ | ☐ | ☐ | ☐ | ☐ | ☐ |

### INSPECTION

| HIVE NUMBER | ① | ② | ③ | ④ | ⑤ | ⑥ |
|---|---|---|---|---|---|---|

### PRODUCTIVITY & REPRODUCTION

| | | | | | | |
|---|---|---|---|---|---|---|
| AMOUNT OF HONEY | | | | | | |
| GENERAL POPULATION | | | | | | |
| AMOUNT OF BROOD | | | | | | |
| AMOUNT OF SPACE | | | | | | |

### BEHAVIOUR & ACTIVITIES

| | | | | | | |
|---|---|---|---|---|---|---|
| USUAL ENTERING AND EXITING ACTIVITY? | | | | | | |
| CALM BEHAVIOUR WHEN OPENING HIVE? | | | | | | |
| BEES BRINGING POLLEN INTO HIVE? | | | | | | |
| SIGNS OF ROBBERY AMONG THE BEES? | | | | | | |

### HEALTH STATUS

| | | | | | | |
|---|---|---|---|---|---|---|
| BEES SEEM WEAK OR LAZY? | | | | | | |
| HIGH AMOUNT OF DEAD BEES? | | | | | | |
| QUEEN BEE IS PRESENT / IDENTIFIABLE? | | | | | | |
| INFESTATION BY ANTS / ANTS PRESENT? | | | | | | |
| INFESTATION BY WAX MOTH / WAX MOTH PRESENT? | | | | | | |
| NEGATIVE ODOUR NOTICEABLE? | | | | | | |

|  | COLONY NAME |
|--|--|
|  | DATE |
|  | TIME |

**WEATHER CONDITIONS**

🌡 _____  ☀  ⛅  🌧  ⛈  ❄
🚩 _____  ☐  ☐  ☐  ☐  ☐

## INSPECTION

| HIVE NUMBER | ① | ② | ③ | ④ | ⑤ | ⑥ |
|---|---|---|---|---|---|---|

### PRODUCTIVITY & REPRODUCTION

| | | | | | | |
|---|---|---|---|---|---|---|
| AMOUNT OF HONEY | | | | | | |
| GENERAL POPULATION | | | | | | |
| AMOUNT OF BROOD | | | | | | |
| AMOUNT OF SPACE | | | | | | |

### BEHAVIOUR & ACTIVITIES

| | | | | | | |
|---|---|---|---|---|---|---|
| USUAL ENTERING AND EXITING ACTIVITY? | | | | | | |
| CALM BEHAVIOUR WHEN OPENING HIVE? | | | | | | |
| BEES BRINGING POLLEN INTO HIVE? | | | | | | |
| SIGNS OF ROBBERY AMONG THE BEES? | | | | | | |

### HEALTH STATUS

| | | | | | | |
|---|---|---|---|---|---|---|
| BEES SEEM WEAK OR LAZY? | | | | | | |
| HIGH AMOUNT OF DEAD BEES? | | | | | | |
| QUEEN BEE IS PRESENT / IDENTIFIABLE? | | | | | | |
| INFESTATION BY ANTS / ANTS PRESENT? | | | | | | |
| INFESTATION BY WAX MOTH / WAX MOTH PRESENT? | | | | | | |
| NEGATIVE ODOUR NOTICEABLE? | | | | | | |

| COLONY NAME | |
|---|---|
| DATE | |
| TIME | |

**WEATHER CONDITIONS**

🌡 _____   ☀ ☁ 🌧 ⛈ ❄
🚩 _____   ☐ ☐ ☐ ☐ ☐

## INSPECTION

| HIVE NUMBER | ① | ② | ③ | ④ | ⑤ | ⑥ |
|---|---|---|---|---|---|---|

## PRODUCTIVITY & REPRODUCTION

| | | | | | | |
|---|---|---|---|---|---|---|
| AMOUNT OF HONEY | | | | | | |
| GENERAL POPULATION | | | | | | |
| AMOUNT OF BROOD | | | | | | |
| AMOUNT OF SPACE | | | | | | |

## BEHAVIOUR & ACTIVITIES

| | | | | | | |
|---|---|---|---|---|---|---|
| USUAL ENTERING AND EXITING ACTIVITY? | | | | | | |
| CALM BEHAVIOUR WHEN OPENING HIVE? | | | | | | |
| BEES BRINGING POLLEN INTO HIVE? | | | | | | |
| SIGNS OF ROBBERY AMONG THE BEES? | | | | | | |

## HEALTH STATUS

| | | | | | | |
|---|---|---|---|---|---|---|
| BEES SEEM WEAK OR LAZY? | | | | | | |
| HIGH AMOUNT OF DEAD BEES? | | | | | | |
| QUEEN BEE IS PRESENT / IDENTIFIABLE? | | | | | | |
| INFESTATION BY ANTS / ANTS PRESENT? | | | | | | |
| INFESTATION BY WAX MOTH / WAX MOTH PRESENT? | | | | | | |
| NEGATIVE ODOUR NOTICEABLE? | | | | | | |

| COLONY NAME | | WEATHER CONDITIONS | | | | | |
|---|---|---|---|---|---|---|---|
| DATE | | 🌡 ___ | ☀ | ⛅ | 🌧 | ⛈ | ❄ |
| TIME | | 🚩 ___ | ☐ | ☐ | ☐ | ☐ | ☐ |

## INSPECTION

| HIVE NUMBER | 1 | 2 | 3 | 4 | 5 | 6 |
|---|---|---|---|---|---|---|

## PRODUCTIVITY & REPRODUCTION

| | 1 | 2 | 3 | 4 | 5 | 6 |
|---|---|---|---|---|---|---|
| AMOUNT OF HONEY | | | | | | |
| GENERAL POPULATION | | | | | | |
| AMOUNT OF BROOD | | | | | | |
| AMOUNT OF SPACE | | | | | | |

## BEHAVIOUR & ACTIVITIES

| | 1 | 2 | 3 | 4 | 5 | 6 |
|---|---|---|---|---|---|---|
| USUAL ENTERING AND EXITING ACTIVITY? | | | | | | |
| CALM BEHAVIOUR WHEN OPENING HIVE? | | | | | | |
| BEES BRINGING POLLEN INTO HIVE? | | | | | | |
| SIGNS OF ROBBERY AMONG THE BEES? | | | | | | |

## HEALTH STATUS

| | 1 | 2 | 3 | 4 | 5 | 6 |
|---|---|---|---|---|---|---|
| BEES SEEM WEAK OR LAZY? | | | | | | |
| HIGH AMOUNT OF DEAD BEES? | | | | | | |
| QUEEN BEE IS PRESENT / IDENTIFIABLE? | | | | | | |
| INFESTATION BY ANTS / ANTS PRESENT? | | | | | | |
| INFESTATION BY WAX MOTH / WAX MOTH PRESENT? | | | | | | |
| NEGATIVE ODOUR NOTICEABLE? | | | | | | |

|  | COLONY NAME |
|---|---|
|  | DATE |
|  | TIME |

**WEATHER CONDITIONS**

🌡 _____ ☀ ⛅ 🌦 ⛈ ❄
🚩 _____ ☐ ☐ ☐ ☐ ☐

## INSPECTION

| HIVE NUMBER | ① | ② | ③ | ④ | ⑤ | ⑥ |
|---|---|---|---|---|---|---|

## PRODUCTIVITY & REPRODUCTION

| | | | | | | |
|---|---|---|---|---|---|---|
| AMOUNT OF HONEY | | | | | | |
| GENERAL POPULATION | | | | | | |
| AMOUNT OF BROOD | | | | | | |
| AMOUNT OF SPACE | | | | | | |

## BEHAVIOUR & ACTIVITIES

| | | | | | | |
|---|---|---|---|---|---|---|
| USUAL ENTERING AND EXITING ACTIVITY? | | | | | | |
| CALM BEHAVIOUR WHEN OPENING HIVE? | | | | | | |
| BEES BRINGING POLLEN INTO HIVE? | | | | | | |
| SIGNS OF ROBBERY AMONG THE BEES? | | | | | | |

## HEALTH STATUS

| | | | | | | |
|---|---|---|---|---|---|---|
| BEES SEEM WEAK OR LAZY? | | | | | | |
| HIGH AMOUNT OF DEAD BEES? | | | | | | |
| QUEEN BEE IS PRESENT / IDENTIFIABLE? | | | | | | |
| INFESTATION BY ANTS / ANTS PRESENT? | | | | | | |
| INFESTATION BY WAX MOTH / WAX MOTH PRESENT? | | | | | | |
| NEGATIVE ODOUR NOTICEABLE? | | | | | | |

| COLONY NAME | | WEATHER CONDITIONS | |
|---|---|---|---|
| DATE | | 🌡 ____ ☀ ⛅ 🌧 ⛈ ❄ | |
| TIME | | 🚩 ____ ☐ ☐ ☐ ☐ ☐ | |

## INSPECTION

| HIVE NUMBER | ① | ② | ③ | ④ | ⑤ | ⑥ |
|---|---|---|---|---|---|---|

## PRODUCTIVITY & REPRODUCTION

| | | | | | | |
|---|---|---|---|---|---|---|
| AMOUNT OF HONEY | | | | | | |
| GENERAL POPULATION | | | | | | |
| AMOUNT OF BROOD | | | | | | |
| AMOUNT OF SPACE | | | | | | |

## BEHAVIOUR & ACTIVITIES

| | | | | | | |
|---|---|---|---|---|---|---|
| USUAL ENTERING AND EXITING ACTIVITY? | | | | | | |
| CALM BEHAVIOUR WHEN OPENING HIVE? | | | | | | |
| BEES BRINGING POLLEN INTO HIVE? | | | | | | |
| SIGNS OF ROBBERY AMONG THE BEES? | | | | | | |

## HEALTH STATUS

| | | | | | | |
|---|---|---|---|---|---|---|
| BEES SEEM WEAK OR LAZY? | | | | | | |
| HIGH AMOUNT OF DEAD BEES? | | | | | | |
| QUEEN BEE IS PRESENT / IDENTIFIABLE? | | | | | | |
| INFESTATION BY ANTS / ANTS PRESENT? | | | | | | |
| INFESTATION BY WAX MOTH / WAX MOTH PRESENT? | | | | | | |
| NEGATIVE ODOUR NOTICEABLE? | | | | | | |

| COLONY NAME | |
|---|---|
| DATE | |
| TIME | |

**WEATHER CONDITIONS**

🌡 _____  ☀ ☁ 🌧 ⛈ ❄
🚩 _____  ☐ ☐ ☐ ☐ ☐

## INSPECTION

| HIVE NUMBER | ① | ② | ③ | ④ | ⑤ | ⑥ |
|---|---|---|---|---|---|---|

## PRODUCTIVITY & REPRODUCTION

| | | | | | | |
|---|---|---|---|---|---|---|
| AMOUNT OF HONEY | | | | | | |
| GENERAL POPULATION | | | | | | |
| AMOUNT OF BROOD | | | | | | |
| AMOUNT OF SPACE | | | | | | |

## BEHAVIOUR & ACTIVITIES

| | | | | | | |
|---|---|---|---|---|---|---|
| USUAL ENTERING AND EXITING ACTIVITY? | | | | | | |
| CALM BEHAVIOUR WHEN OPENING HIVE? | | | | | | |
| BEES BRINGING POLLEN INTO HIVE? | | | | | | |
| SIGNS OF ROBBERY AMONG THE BEES? | | | | | | |

## HEALTH STATUS

| | | | | | | |
|---|---|---|---|---|---|---|
| BEES SEEM WEAK OR LAZY? | | | | | | |
| HIGH AMOUNT OF DEAD BEES? | | | | | | |
| QUEEN BEE IS PRESENT / IDENTIFIABLE? | | | | | | |
| INFESTATION BY ANTS / ANTS PRESENT? | | | | | | |
| INFESTATION BY WAX MOTH / WAX MOTH PRESENT? | | | | | | |
| NEGATIVE ODOUR NOTICEABLE? | | | | | | |

| | COLONY NAME | |
|---|---|---|
| | DATE | |
| | TIME | |

**WEATHER CONDITIONS**

🌡 ____   ☀ ☁ 🌧 ⛈ ❄
🚩 ____   ☐ ☐ ☐ ☐ ☐

## INSPECTION

| HIVE NUMBER | 1 | 2 | 3 | 4 | 5 | 6 |
|---|---|---|---|---|---|---|

## PRODUCTIVITY & REPRODUCTION

| | | | | | | |
|---|---|---|---|---|---|---|
| AMOUNT OF HONEY | | | | | | |
| GENERAL POPULATION | | | | | | |
| AMOUNT OF BROOD | | | | | | |
| AMOUNT OF SPACE | | | | | | |

## BEHAVIOUR & ACTIVITIES

| | | | | | | |
|---|---|---|---|---|---|---|
| USUAL ENTERING AND EXITING ACTIVITY? | | | | | | |
| CALM BEHAVIOUR WHEN OPENING HIVE? | | | | | | |
| BEES BRINGING POLLEN INTO HIVE? | | | | | | |
| SIGNS OF ROBBERY AMONG THE BEES? | | | | | | |

## HEALTH STATUS

| | | | | | | |
|---|---|---|---|---|---|---|
| BEES SEEM WEAK OR LAZY? | | | | | | |
| HIGH AMOUNT OF DEAD BEES? | | | | | | |
| QUEEN BEE IS PRESENT / IDENTIFIABLE? | | | | | | |
| INFESTATION BY ANTS / ANTS PRESENT? | | | | | | |
| INFESTATION BY WAX MOTH / WAX MOTH PRESENT? | | | | | | |
| NEGATIVE ODOUR NOTICEABLE? | | | | | | |

|  | COLONY NAME |
|---|---|
|  | DATE |
|  | TIME |

**WEATHER CONDITIONS**

🌡 ____   ☀ ☁ 🌧 ⛈ ❄
🚩 ____   ☐ ☐ ☐ ☐ ☐

## INSPECTION

| HIVE NUMBER | ① | ② | ③ | ④ | ⑤ | ⑥ |
|---|---|---|---|---|---|---|

## PRODUCTIVITY & REPRODUCTION

| | | | | | | |
|---|---|---|---|---|---|---|
| AMOUNT OF HONEY | | | | | | |
| GENERAL POPULATION | | | | | | |
| AMOUNT OF BROOD | | | | | | |
| AMOUNT OF SPACE | | | | | | |

## BEHAVIOUR & ACTIVITIES

| | | | | | | |
|---|---|---|---|---|---|---|
| USUAL ENTERING AND EXITING ACTIVITY? | | | | | | |
| CALM BEHAVIOUR WHEN OPENING HIVE? | | | | | | |
| BEES BRINGING POLLEN INTO HIVE? | | | | | | |
| SIGNS OF ROBBERY AMONG THE BEES? | | | | | | |

## HEALTH STATUS

| | | | | | | |
|---|---|---|---|---|---|---|
| BEES SEEM WEAK OR LAZY? | | | | | | |
| HIGH AMOUNT OF DEAD BEES? | | | | | | |
| QUEEN BEE IS PRESENT / IDENTIFIABLE? | | | | | | |
| INFESTATION BY ANTS / ANTS PRESENT? | | | | | | |
| INFESTATION BY WAX MOTH / WAX MOTH PRESENT? | | | | | | |
| NEGATIVE ODOUR NOTICEABLE? | | | | | | |

| | COLONY NAME |
|---|---|
| | DATE |
| | TIME |

## WEATHER CONDITIONS

🌡 _____  ☀  ⛅  🌧  ⛈  ❄
🚩 _____  ☐  ☐  ☐  ☐  ☐

### INSPECTION

| HIVE NUMBER | ① | ② | ③ | ④ | ⑤ | ⑥ |
|---|---|---|---|---|---|---|

### PRODUCTIVITY & REPRODUCTION

| | | | | | | |
|---|---|---|---|---|---|---|
| AMOUNT OF HONEY | | | | | | |
| GENERAL POPULATION | | | | | | |
| AMOUNT OF BROOD | | | | | | |
| AMOUNT OF SPACE | | | | | | |

### BEHAVIOUR & ACTIVITIES

| | | | | | | |
|---|---|---|---|---|---|---|
| USUAL ENTERING AND EXITING ACTIVITY? | | | | | | |
| CALM BEHAVIOUR WHEN OPENING HIVE? | | | | | | |
| BEES BRINGING POLLEN INTO HIVE? | | | | | | |
| SIGNS OF ROBBERY AMONG THE BEES? | | | | | | |

### HEALTH STATUS

| | | | | | | |
|---|---|---|---|---|---|---|
| BEES SEEM WEAK OR LAZY? | | | | | | |
| HIGH AMOUNT OF DEAD BEES? | | | | | | |
| QUEEN BEE IS PRESENT / IDENTIFIABLE? | | | | | | |
| INFESTATION BY ANTS / ANTS PRESENT? | | | | | | |
| INFESTATION BY WAX MOTH / WAX MOTH PRESENT? | | | | | | |
| NEGATIVE ODOUR NOTICEABLE? | | | | | | |

|  |  |
|---|---|
| 🏠 COLONY NAME | |
| 📅 DATE | |
| 🕐 TIME | |

**WEATHER CONDITIONS**

🌡 _____   ☀  ⛅  🌧  ⛈  ❄
🚩 _____   ☐  ☐  ☐  ☐  ☐

## INSPECTION

| HIVE NUMBER | 1 | 2 | 3 | 4 | 5 | 6 |
|---|---|---|---|---|---|---|

## PRODUCTIVITY & REPRODUCTION

| | | | | | | |
|---|---|---|---|---|---|---|
| AMOUNT OF HONEY | | | | | | |
| GENERAL POPULATION | | | | | | |
| AMOUNT OF BROOD | | | | | | |
| AMOUNT OF SPACE | | | | | | |

## BEHAVIOUR & ACTIVITIES

| | | | | | | |
|---|---|---|---|---|---|---|
| USUAL ENTERING AND EXITING ACTIVITY? | | | | | | |
| CALM BEHAVIOUR WHEN OPENING HIVE? | | | | | | |
| BEES BRINGING POLLEN INTO HIVE? | | | | | | |
| SIGNS OF ROBBERY AMONG THE BEES? | | | | | | |

## HEALTH STATUS

| | | | | | | |
|---|---|---|---|---|---|---|
| BEES SEEM WEAK OR LAZY? | | | | | | |
| HIGH AMOUNT OF DEAD BEES? | | | | | | |
| QUEEN BEE IS PRESENT / IDENTIFIABLE? | | | | | | |
| INFESTATION BY ANTS / ANTS PRESENT? | | | | | | |
| INFESTATION BY WAX MOTH / WAX MOTH PRESENT? | | | | | | |
| NEGATIVE ODOUR NOTICEABLE? | | | | | | |

|  | COLONY NAME |
|---|---|
|  | DATE |
|  | TIME |

## WEATHER CONDITIONS

🌡 _____  ☀  ⛅  🌧  ⛈  ❄
🚩 _____  ☐  ☐  ☐  ☐  ☐

## INSPECTION

| HIVE NUMBER | 1 | 2 | 3 | 4 | 5 | 6 |
|---|---|---|---|---|---|---|

## PRODUCTIVITY & REPRODUCTION

| | | | | | | |
|---|---|---|---|---|---|---|
| AMOUNT OF HONEY | | | | | | |
| GENERAL POPULATION | | | | | | |
| AMOUNT OF BROOD | | | | | | |
| AMOUNT OF SPACE | | | | | | |

## BEHAVIOUR & ACTIVITIES

| | | | | | | |
|---|---|---|---|---|---|---|
| USUAL ENTERING AND EXITING ACTIVITY? | | | | | | |
| CALM BEHAVIOUR WHEN OPENING HIVE? | | | | | | |
| BEES BRINGING POLLEN INTO HIVE? | | | | | | |
| SIGNS OF ROBBERY AMONG THE BEES? | | | | | | |

## HEALTH STATUS

| | | | | | | |
|---|---|---|---|---|---|---|
| BEES SEEM WEAK OR LAZY? | | | | | | |
| HIGH AMOUNT OF DEAD BEES? | | | | | | |
| QUEEN BEE IS PRESENT / IDENTIFIABLE? | | | | | | |
| INFESTATION BY ANTS / ANTS PRESENT? | | | | | | |
| INFESTATION BY WAX MOTH / WAX MOTH PRESENT? | | | | | | |
| NEGATIVE ODOUR NOTICEABLE? | | | | | | |

| COLONY NAME | |
|---|---|
| DATE | |
| TIME | |

## WEATHER CONDITIONS

🌡 _____  ☀ ⛅ 🌧 ⛈ ❄
🚩 _____  ☐ ☐ ☐ ☐ ☐

## INSPECTION

| HIVE NUMBER | ① | ② | ③ | ④ | ⑤ | ⑥ |
|---|---|---|---|---|---|---|

## PRODUCTIVITY & REPRODUCTION

| | | | | | | |
|---|---|---|---|---|---|---|
| AMOUNT OF HONEY | | | | | | |
| GENERAL POPULATION | | | | | | |
| AMOUNT OF BROOD | | | | | | |
| AMOUNT OF SPACE | | | | | | |

## BEHAVIOUR & ACTIVITIES

| | | | | | | |
|---|---|---|---|---|---|---|
| USUAL ENTERING AND EXITING ACTIVITY? | | | | | | |
| CALM BEHAVIOUR WHEN OPENING HIVE? | | | | | | |
| BEES BRINGING POLLEN INTO HIVE? | | | | | | |
| SIGNS OF ROBBERY AMONG THE BEES? | | | | | | |

## HEALTH STATUS

| | | | | | | |
|---|---|---|---|---|---|---|
| BEES SEEM WEAK OR LAZY? | | | | | | |
| HIGH AMOUNT OF DEAD BEES? | | | | | | |
| QUEEN BEE IS PRESENT / IDENTIFIABLE? | | | | | | |
| INFESTATION BY ANTS / ANTS PRESENT? | | | | | | |
| INFESTATION BY WAX MOTH / WAX MOTH PRESENT? | | | | | | |
| NEGATIVE ODOUR NOTICEABLE? | | | | | | |

| | COLONY NAME |
|---|---|
| | DATE |
| | TIME |

**WEATHER CONDITIONS**

🌡 _____  ☀️  ⛅  🌧  ⛈  ❄️
🚩 _____  ☐   ☐   ☐   ☐   ☐

## INSPECTION

| HIVE NUMBER | ① | ② | ③ | ④ | ⑤ | ⑥ |
|---|---|---|---|---|---|---|

## PRODUCTIVITY & REPRODUCTION

| | | | | | | |
|---|---|---|---|---|---|---|
| AMOUNT OF HONEY | | | | | | |
| GENERAL POPULATION | | | | | | |
| AMOUNT OF BROOD | | | | | | |
| AMOUNT OF SPACE | | | | | | |

## BEHAVIOUR & ACTIVITIES

| | | | | | | |
|---|---|---|---|---|---|---|
| USUAL ENTERING AND EXITING ACTIVITY? | | | | | | |
| CALM BEHAVIOUR WHEN OPENING HIVE? | | | | | | |
| BEES BRINGING POLLEN INTO HIVE? | | | | | | |
| SIGNS OF ROBBERY AMONG THE BEES? | | | | | | |

## HEALTH STATUS

| | | | | | | |
|---|---|---|---|---|---|---|
| BEES SEEM WEAK OR LAZY? | | | | | | |
| HIGH AMOUNT OF DEAD BEES? | | | | | | |
| QUEEN BEE IS PRESENT / IDENTIFIABLE? | | | | | | |
| INFESTATION BY ANTS / ANTS PRESENT? | | | | | | |
| INFESTATION BY WAX MOTH / WAX MOTH PRESENT? | | | | | | |
| NEGATIVE ODOUR NOTICEABLE? | | | | | | |

| COLONY NAME | | WEATHER CONDITIONS | |
|---|---|---|---|
| DATE | | 🌡 ___ ☀ ⛅ 🌧 ⛈ ❄ | |
| TIME | | 🚩 ___ ☐ ☐ ☐ ☐ ☐ | |

## INSPECTION

| HIVE NUMBER | 1 | 2 | 3 | 4 | 5 | 6 |
|---|---|---|---|---|---|---|

## PRODUCTIVITY & REPRODUCTION

| | 1 | 2 | 3 | 4 | 5 | 6 |
|---|---|---|---|---|---|---|
| AMOUNT OF HONEY | | | | | | |
| GENERAL POPULATION | | | | | | |
| AMOUNT OF BROOD | | | | | | |
| AMOUNT OF SPACE | | | | | | |

## BEHAVIOUR & ACTIVITIES

| | 1 | 2 | 3 | 4 | 5 | 6 |
|---|---|---|---|---|---|---|
| USUAL ENTERING AND EXITING ACTIVITY? | | | | | | |
| CALM BEHAVIOUR WHEN OPENING HIVE? | | | | | | |
| BEES BRINGING POLLEN INTO HIVE? | | | | | | |
| SIGNS OF ROBBERY AMONG THE BEES? | | | | | | |

## HEALTH STATUS

| | 1 | 2 | 3 | 4 | 5 | 6 |
|---|---|---|---|---|---|---|
| BEES SEEM WEAK OR LAZY? | | | | | | |
| HIGH AMOUNT OF DEAD BEES? | | | | | | |
| QUEEN BEE IS PRESENT / IDENTIFIABLE? | | | | | | |
| INFESTATION BY ANTS / ANTS PRESENT? | | | | | | |
| INFESTATION BY WAX MOTH / WAX MOTH PRESENT? | | | | | | |
| NEGATIVE ODOUR NOTICEABLE? | | | | | | |

| COLONY NAME | |
|---|---|
| DATE | |
| TIME | |

**WEATHER CONDITIONS**

| 🌡 ___ | ☀ ☐ | ⛅ ☐ | 🌦 ☐ | ⛈ ☐ | ❄ ☐ |
|---|---|---|---|---|---|
| 🚩 ___ | | | | | |

## INSPECTION

| HIVE NUMBER | ① | ② | ③ | ④ | ⑤ | ⑥ |
|---|---|---|---|---|---|---|

### PRODUCTIVITY & REPRODUCTION

| | | | | | | |
|---|---|---|---|---|---|---|
| AMOUNT OF HONEY | | | | | | |
| GENERAL POPULATION | | | | | | |
| AMOUNT OF BROOD | | | | | | |
| AMOUNT OF SPACE | | | | | | |

### BEHAVIOUR & ACTIVITIES

| | | | | | | |
|---|---|---|---|---|---|---|
| USUAL ENTERING AND EXITING ACTIVITY? | | | | | | |
| CALM BEHAVIOUR WHEN OPENING HIVE? | | | | | | |
| BEES BRINGING POLLEN INTO HIVE? | | | | | | |
| SIGNS OF ROBBERY AMONG THE BEES? | | | | | | |

### HEALTH STATUS

| | | | | | | |
|---|---|---|---|---|---|---|
| BEES SEEM WEAK OR LAZY? | | | | | | |
| HIGH AMOUNT OF DEAD BEES? | | | | | | |
| QUEEN BEE IS PRESENT / IDENTIFIABLE? | | | | | | |
| INFESTATION BY ANTS / ANTS PRESENT? | | | | | | |
| INFESTATION BY WAX MOTH / WAX MOTH PRESENT? | | | | | | |
| NEGATIVE ODOUR NOTICEABLE? | | | | | | |

|  |  |
|---|---|
| 🏠 **COLONY NAME** | |
| 📅 **DATE** | |
| 🕐 **TIME** | |

### WEATHER CONDITIONS

🌡️ _____  ☀️  ⛅  🌧️  ⛈️  ❄️
🚩 _____  ☐  ☐  ☐  ☐  ☐

### INSPECTION

| HIVE NUMBER | ① | ② | ③ | ④ | ⑤ | ⑥ |
|---|---|---|---|---|---|---|

### PRODUCTIVITY & REPRODUCTION

| | | | | | | |
|---|---|---|---|---|---|---|
| AMOUNT OF HONEY | | | | | | |
| GENERAL POPULATION | | | | | | |
| AMOUNT OF BROOD | | | | | | |
| AMOUNT OF SPACE | | | | | | |

### BEHAVIOUR & ACTIVITIES

| | | | | | | |
|---|---|---|---|---|---|---|
| USUAL ENTERING AND EXITING ACTIVITY? | | | | | | |
| CALM BEHAVIOUR WHEN OPENING HIVE? | | | | | | |
| BEES BRINGING POLLEN INTO HIVE? | | | | | | |
| SIGNS OF ROBBERY AMONG THE BEES? | | | | | | |

### HEALTH STATUS

| | | | | | | |
|---|---|---|---|---|---|---|
| BEES SEEM WEAK OR LAZY? | | | | | | |
| HIGH AMOUNT OF DEAD BEES? | | | | | | |
| QUEEN BEE IS PRESENT / IDENTIFIABLE? | | | | | | |
| INFESTATION BY ANTS / ANTS PRESENT? | | | | | | |
| INFESTATION BY WAX MOTH / WAX MOTH PRESENT? | | | | | | |
| NEGATIVE ODOUR NOTICEABLE? | | | | | | |

|  | COLONY NAME |
|---|---|
|  | DATE |
|  | TIME |

### WEATHER CONDITIONS

| 🌡 | ___ | ☀ | ⛅ | 🌧 | ⛈ | ❄ |
|---|---|---|---|---|---|---|
| 🚩 | ___ |  | ☐ | ☐ | ☐ | ☐ |

### INSPECTION

| HIVE NUMBER | 1 | 2 | 3 | 4 | 5 | 6 |
|---|---|---|---|---|---|---|

### PRODUCTIVITY & REPRODUCTION

| | | | | | | |
|---|---|---|---|---|---|---|
| AMOUNT OF HONEY | | | | | | |
| GENERAL POPULATION | | | | | | |
| AMOUNT OF BROOD | | | | | | |
| AMOUNT OF SPACE | | | | | | |

### BEHAVIOUR & ACTIVITIES

| | | | | | | |
|---|---|---|---|---|---|---|
| USUAL ENTERING AND EXITING ACTIVITY? | | | | | | |
| CALM BEHAVIOUR WHEN OPENING HIVE? | | | | | | |
| BEES BRINGING POLLEN INTO HIVE? | | | | | | |
| SIGNS OF ROBBERY AMONG THE BEES? | | | | | | |

### HEALTH STATUS

| | | | | | | |
|---|---|---|---|---|---|---|
| BEES SEEM WEAK OR LAZY? | | | | | | |
| HIGH AMOUNT OF DEAD BEES? | | | | | | |
| QUEEN BEE IS PRESENT / IDENTIFIABLE? | | | | | | |
| INFESTATION BY ANTS / ANTS PRESENT? | | | | | | |
| INFESTATION BY WAX MOTH / WAX MOTH PRESENT? | | | | | | |
| NEGATIVE ODOUR NOTICEABLE? | | | | | | |

|  | COLONY NAME |
|---|---|
|  | DATE |
|  | TIME |

**WEATHER CONDITIONS**

🌡 _____   ☀ ☁ 🌧 ⛈ ❄
🚩 _____   ☐ ☐ ☐ ☐ ☐

## INSPECTION

| HIVE NUMBER | 1 | 2 | 3 | 4 | 5 | 6 |
|---|---|---|---|---|---|---|

## PRODUCTIVITY & REPRODUCTION

| | | | | | | |
|---|---|---|---|---|---|---|
| AMOUNT OF HONEY | | | | | | |
| GENERAL POPULATION | | | | | | |
| AMOUNT OF BROOD | | | | | | |
| AMOUNT OF SPACE | | | | | | |

## BEHAVIOUR & ACTIVITIES

| | | | | | | |
|---|---|---|---|---|---|---|
| USUAL ENTERING AND EXITING ACTIVITY? | | | | | | |
| CALM BEHAVIOUR WHEN OPENING HIVE? | | | | | | |
| BEES BRINGING POLLEN INTO HIVE? | | | | | | |
| SIGNS OF ROBBERY AMONG THE BEES? | | | | | | |

## HEALTH STATUS

| | | | | | | |
|---|---|---|---|---|---|---|
| BEES SEEM WEAK OR LAZY? | | | | | | |
| HIGH AMOUNT OF DEAD BEES? | | | | | | |
| QUEEN BEE IS PRESENT / IDENTIFIABLE? | | | | | | |
| INFESTATION BY ANTS / ANTS PRESENT? | | | | | | |
| INFESTATION BY WAX MOTH / WAX MOTH PRESENT? | | | | | | |
| NEGATIVE ODOUR NOTICEABLE? | | | | | | |

|  | COLONY NAME |
|---|---|
|  | DATE |
|  | TIME |

| WEATHER CONDITIONS | | | | | |
|---|---|---|---|---|---|
| 🌡 ——— | ☀ | ⛅ | 🌧 | ⛈ | ❄ |
| 🚩 ——— | ☐ | ☐ | ☐ | ☐ | ☐ |

## INSPECTION

| HIVE NUMBER | 1 | 2 | 3 | 4 | 5 | 6 |
|---|---|---|---|---|---|---|

### PRODUCTIVITY & REPRODUCTION

| | 1 | 2 | 3 | 4 | 5 | 6 |
|---|---|---|---|---|---|---|
| AMOUNT OF HONEY | | | | | | |
| GENERAL POPULATION | | | | | | |
| AMOUNT OF BROOD | | | | | | |
| AMOUNT OF SPACE | | | | | | |

### BEHAVIOUR & ACTIVITIES

| | 1 | 2 | 3 | 4 | 5 | 6 |
|---|---|---|---|---|---|---|
| USUAL ENTERING AND EXITING ACTIVITY? | | | | | | |
| CALM BEHAVIOUR WHEN OPENING HIVE? | | | | | | |
| BEES BRINGING POLLEN INTO HIVE? | | | | | | |
| SIGNS OF ROBBERY AMONG THE BEES? | | | | | | |

### HEALTH STATUS

| | 1 | 2 | 3 | 4 | 5 | 6 |
|---|---|---|---|---|---|---|
| BEES SEEM WEAK OR LAZY? | | | | | | |
| HIGH AMOUNT OF DEAD BEES? | | | | | | |
| QUEEN BEE IS PRESENT / IDENTIFIABLE? | | | | | | |
| INFESTATION BY ANTS / ANTS PRESENT? | | | | | | |
| INFESTATION BY WAX MOTH / WAX MOTH PRESENT? | | | | | | |
| NEGATIVE ODOUR NOTICEABLE? | | | | | | |

|  | COLONY NAME |
|---|---|
|  | DATE |
|  | TIME |

## WEATHER CONDITIONS

🌡 ____  ☀ ☁ 🌧 ⛈ ❄
🚩 ____  ☐ ☐ ☐ ☐ ☐

## INSPECTION

| HIVE NUMBER | 1 | 2 | 3 | 4 | 5 | 6 |
|---|---|---|---|---|---|---|

## PRODUCTIVITY & REPRODUCTION

| | 1 | 2 | 3 | 4 | 5 | 6 |
|---|---|---|---|---|---|---|
| AMOUNT OF HONEY | | | | | | |
| GENERAL POPULATION | | | | | | |
| AMOUNT OF BROOD | | | | | | |
| AMOUNT OF SPACE | | | | | | |

## BEHAVIOUR & ACTIVITIES

| | 1 | 2 | 3 | 4 | 5 | 6 |
|---|---|---|---|---|---|---|
| USUAL ENTERING AND EXITING ACTIVITY? | | | | | | |
| CALM BEHAVIOUR WHEN OPENING HIVE? | | | | | | |
| BEES BRINGING POLLEN INTO HIVE? | | | | | | |
| SIGNS OF ROBBERY AMONG THE BEES? | | | | | | |

## HEALTH STATUS

| | 1 | 2 | 3 | 4 | 5 | 6 |
|---|---|---|---|---|---|---|
| BEES SEEM WEAK OR LAZY? | | | | | | |
| HIGH AMOUNT OF DEAD BEES? | | | | | | |
| QUEEN BEE IS PRESENT / IDENTIFIABLE? | | | | | | |
| INFESTATION BY ANTS / ANTS PRESENT? | | | | | | |
| INFESTATION BY WAX MOTH / WAX MOTH PRESENT? | | | | | | |
| NEGATIVE ODOUR NOTICEABLE? | | | | | | |

|  | COLONY NAME |
|---|---|
|  | DATE |
|  | TIME |

## WEATHER CONDITIONS

🌡 ____  ☀ ☁ 🌧 ⛈ ❄
🚩 ____  ☐ ☐ ☐ ☐ ☐

## INSPECTION

| HIVE NUMBER | ① | ② | ③ | ④ | ⑤ | ⑥ |
|---|---|---|---|---|---|---|

## PRODUCTIVITY & REPRODUCTION

| | | | | | | |
|---|---|---|---|---|---|---|
| AMOUNT OF HONEY | | | | | | |
| GENERAL POPULATION | | | | | | |
| AMOUNT OF BROOD | | | | | | |
| AMOUNT OF SPACE | | | | | | |

## BEHAVIOUR & ACTIVITIES

| | | | | | | |
|---|---|---|---|---|---|---|
| USUAL ENTERING AND EXITING ACTIVITY? | | | | | | |
| CALM BEHAVIOUR WHEN OPENING HIVE? | | | | | | |
| BEES BRINGING POLLEN INTO HIVE? | | | | | | |
| SIGNS OF ROBBERY AMONG THE BEES? | | | | | | |

## HEALTH STATUS

| | | | | | | |
|---|---|---|---|---|---|---|
| BEES SEEM WEAK OR LAZY? | | | | | | |
| HIGH AMOUNT OF DEAD BEES? | | | | | | |
| QUEEN BEE IS PRESENT / IDENTIFIABLE? | | | | | | |
| INFESTATION BY ANTS / ANTS PRESENT? | | | | | | |
| INFESTATION BY WAX MOTH / WAX MOTH PRESENT? | | | | | | |
| NEGATIVE ODOUR NOTICEABLE? | | | | | | |

| COLONY NAME | |
|---|---|
| DATE | |
| TIME | |

### WEATHER CONDITIONS

🌡 _____  ☀  ⛅  🌧  ⛈  ❄
🚩 _____  ☐  ☐  ☐  ☐  ☐

## INSPECTION

| HIVE NUMBER | ① | ② | ③ | ④ | ⑤ | ⑥ |
|---|---|---|---|---|---|---|

### PRODUCTIVITY & REPRODUCTION

| | | | | | | |
|---|---|---|---|---|---|---|
| AMOUNT OF HONEY | | | | | | |
| GENERAL POPULATION | | | | | | |
| AMOUNT OF BROOD | | | | | | |
| AMOUNT OF SPACE | | | | | | |

### BEHAVIOUR & ACTIVITIES

| | | | | | | |
|---|---|---|---|---|---|---|
| USUAL ENTERING AND EXITING ACTIVITY? | | | | | | |
| CALM BEHAVIOUR WHEN OPENING HIVE? | | | | | | |
| BEES BRINGING POLLEN INTO HIVE? | | | | | | |
| SIGNS OF ROBBERY AMONG THE BEES? | | | | | | |

### HEALTH STATUS

| | | | | | | |
|---|---|---|---|---|---|---|
| BEES SEEM WEAK OR LAZY? | | | | | | |
| HIGH AMOUNT OF DEAD BEES? | | | | | | |
| QUEEN BEE IS PRESENT / IDENTIFIABLE? | | | | | | |
| INFESTATION BY ANTS / ANTS PRESENT? | | | | | | |
| INFESTATION BY WAX MOTH / WAX MOTH PRESENT? | | | | | | |
| NEGATIVE ODOUR NOTICEABLE? | | | | | | |

| COLONY NAME | |
|---|---|
| DATE | |
| TIME | |

**WEATHER CONDITIONS**

🌡 _____  ☀  ⛅  🌧  ⛈  ❄
🚩 _____  ☐  ☐  ☐  ☐  ☐

## INSPECTION

| HIVE NUMBER | ① | ② | ③ | ④ | ⑤ | ⑥ |
|---|---|---|---|---|---|---|

## PRODUCTIVITY & REPRODUCTION

| | | | | | | |
|---|---|---|---|---|---|---|
| AMOUNT OF HONEY | | | | | | |
| GENERAL POPULATION | | | | | | |
| AMOUNT OF BROOD | | | | | | |
| AMOUNT OF SPACE | | | | | | |

## BEHAVIOUR & ACTIVITIES

| | | | | | | |
|---|---|---|---|---|---|---|
| USUAL ENTERING AND EXITING ACTIVITY? | | | | | | |
| CALM BEHAVIOUR WHEN OPENING HIVE? | | | | | | |
| BEES BRINGING POLLEN INTO HIVE? | | | | | | |
| SIGNS OF ROBBERY AMONG THE BEES? | | | | | | |

## HEALTH STATUS

| | | | | | | |
|---|---|---|---|---|---|---|
| BEES SEEM WEAK OR LAZY? | | | | | | |
| HIGH AMOUNT OF DEAD BEES? | | | | | | |
| QUEEN BEE IS PRESENT / IDENTIFIABLE? | | | | | | |
| INFESTATION BY ANTS / ANTS PRESENT? | | | | | | |
| INFESTATION BY WAX MOTH / WAX MOTH PRESENT? | | | | | | |
| NEGATIVE ODOUR NOTICEABLE? | | | | | | |

| COLONY NAME | |
|---|---|
| DATE | |
| TIME | |

| WEATHER CONDITIONS | | | | | | |
|---|---|---|---|---|---|---|
| 🌡 ___ | ☀ | ⛅ | 🌧 | ⛈ | ❄ | |
| 🚩 ___ | ☐ | ☐ | ☐ | ☐ | ☐ | |

## INSPECTION

| HIVE NUMBER | 1 | 2 | 3 | 4 | 5 | 6 |
|---|---|---|---|---|---|---|

## PRODUCTIVITY & REPRODUCTION

| | 1 | 2 | 3 | 4 | 5 | 6 |
|---|---|---|---|---|---|---|
| AMOUNT OF HONEY | | | | | | |
| GENERAL POPULATION | | | | | | |
| AMOUNT OF BROOD | | | | | | |
| AMOUNT OF SPACE | | | | | | |

## BEHAVIOUR & ACTIVITIES

| | 1 | 2 | 3 | 4 | 5 | 6 |
|---|---|---|---|---|---|---|
| USUAL ENTERING AND EXITING ACTIVITY? | | | | | | |
| CALM BEHAVIOUR WHEN OPENING HIVE? | | | | | | |
| BEES BRINGING POLLEN INTO HIVE? | | | | | | |
| SIGNS OF ROBBERY AMONG THE BEES? | | | | | | |

## HEALTH STATUS

| | 1 | 2 | 3 | 4 | 5 | 6 |
|---|---|---|---|---|---|---|
| BEES SEEM WEAK OR LAZY? | | | | | | |
| HIGH AMOUNT OF DEAD BEES? | | | | | | |
| QUEEN BEE IS PRESENT / IDENTIFIABLE? | | | | | | |
| INFESTATION BY ANTS / ANTS PRESENT? | | | | | | |
| INFESTATION BY WAX MOTH / WAX MOTH PRESENT? | | | | | | |
| NEGATIVE ODOUR NOTICEABLE? | | | | | | |

|  | COLONY NAME |
|---|---|
|  | DATE |
|  | TIME |

**WEATHER CONDITIONS**

🌡 ____ ☀ ⛅ 🌧 ⛈ ❄
🚩 ____ ☐ ☐ ☐ ☐ ☐

## INSPECTION

| HIVE NUMBER | ① | ② | ③ | ④ | ⑤ | ⑥ |
|---|---|---|---|---|---|---|

### PRODUCTIVITY & REPRODUCTION

| | | | | | | |
|---|---|---|---|---|---|---|
| AMOUNT OF HONEY | | | | | | |
| GENERAL POPULATION | | | | | | |
| AMOUNT OF BROOD | | | | | | |
| AMOUNT OF SPACE | | | | | | |

### BEHAVIOUR & ACTIVITIES

| | | | | | | |
|---|---|---|---|---|---|---|
| USUAL ENTERING AND EXITING ACTIVITY? | | | | | | |
| CALM BEHAVIOUR WHEN OPENING HIVE? | | | | | | |
| BEES BRINGING POLLEN INTO HIVE? | | | | | | |
| SIGNS OF ROBBERY AMONG THE BEES? | | | | | | |

### HEALTH STATUS

| | | | | | | |
|---|---|---|---|---|---|---|
| BEES SEEM WEAK OR LAZY? | | | | | | |
| HIGH AMOUNT OF DEAD BEES? | | | | | | |
| QUEEN BEE IS PRESENT / IDENTIFIABLE? | | | | | | |
| INFESTATION BY ANTS / ANTS PRESENT? | | | | | | |
| INFESTATION BY WAX MOTH / WAX MOTH PRESENT? | | | | | | |
| NEGATIVE ODOUR NOTICEABLE? | | | | | | |

| COLONY NAME | | WEATHER CONDITIONS | | | | | |
|---|---|---|---|---|---|---|---|
| DATE | | 🌡 ___ | ☀ ☐ | ⛅ ☐ | 🌧 ☐ | ⛈ ☐ | ❄ ☐ |
| TIME | | 🚩 ___ | | | | | |

## INSPECTION

| HIVE NUMBER | ① | ② | ③ | ④ | ⑤ | ⑥ |
|---|---|---|---|---|---|---|

## PRODUCTIVITY & REPRODUCTION

| | | | | | | |
|---|---|---|---|---|---|---|
| AMOUNT OF HONEY | | | | | | |
| GENERAL POPULATION | | | | | | |
| AMOUNT OF BROOD | | | | | | |
| AMOUNT OF SPACE | | | | | | |

## BEHAVIOUR & ACTIVITIES

| | | | | | | |
|---|---|---|---|---|---|---|
| USUAL ENTERING AND EXITING ACTIVITY? | | | | | | |
| CALM BEHAVIOUR WHEN OPENING HIVE? | | | | | | |
| BEES BRINGING POLLEN INTO HIVE? | | | | | | |
| SIGNS OF ROBBERY AMONG THE BEES? | | | | | | |

## HEALTH STATUS

| | | | | | | |
|---|---|---|---|---|---|---|
| BEES SEEM WEAK OR LAZY? | | | | | | |
| HIGH AMOUNT OF DEAD BEES? | | | | | | |
| QUEEN BEE IS PRESENT / IDENTIFIABLE? | | | | | | |
| INFESTATION BY ANTS / ANTS PRESENT? | | | | | | |
| INFESTATION BY WAX MOTH / WAX MOTH PRESENT? | | | | | | |
| NEGATIVE ODOUR NOTICEABLE? | | | | | | |

|  | COLONY NAME |
|---|---|
|  | DATE |
|  | TIME |

**WEATHER CONDITIONS**

🌡 _____  ☀ ☁ 🌧 ⛈ ❄
💨 _____  ☐ ☐ ☐ ☐ ☐

## INSPECTION

| HIVE NUMBER | ① | ② | ③ | ④ | ⑤ | ⑥ |
|---|---|---|---|---|---|---|

## PRODUCTIVITY & REPRODUCTION

| | | | | | | |
|---|---|---|---|---|---|---|
| AMOUNT OF HONEY | | | | | | |
| GENERAL POPULATION | | | | | | |
| AMOUNT OF BROOD | | | | | | |
| AMOUNT OF SPACE | | | | | | |

## BEHAVIOUR & ACTIVITIES

| | | | | | | |
|---|---|---|---|---|---|---|
| USUAL ENTERING AND EXITING ACTIVITY? | | | | | | |
| CALM BEHAVIOUR WHEN OPENING HIVE? | | | | | | |
| BEES BRINGING POLLEN INTO HIVE? | | | | | | |
| SIGNS OF ROBBERY AMONG THE BEES? | | | | | | |

## HEALTH STATUS

| | | | | | | |
|---|---|---|---|---|---|---|
| BEES SEEM WEAK OR LAZY? | | | | | | |
| HIGH AMOUNT OF DEAD BEES? | | | | | | |
| QUEEN BEE IS PRESENT / IDENTIFIABLE? | | | | | | |
| INFESTATION BY ANTS / ANTS PRESENT? | | | | | | |
| INFESTATION BY WAX MOTH / WAX MOTH PRESENT? | | | | | | |
| NEGATIVE ODOUR NOTICEABLE? | | | | | | |

|  | COLONY NAME |
|---|---|
|  | DATE |
|  | TIME |

**WEATHER CONDITIONS**

Temperature: ____  ☀ ⛅ 🌧 ⛈ ❄
Wind: ____  ☐ ☐ ☐ ☐ ☐

## INSPECTION

| HIVE NUMBER | 1 | 2 | 3 | 4 | 5 | 6 |
|---|---|---|---|---|---|---|

## PRODUCTIVITY & REPRODUCTION

| | | | | | | |
|---|---|---|---|---|---|---|
| AMOUNT OF HONEY | | | | | | |
| GENERAL POPULATION | | | | | | |
| AMOUNT OF BROOD | | | | | | |
| AMOUNT OF SPACE | | | | | | |

## BEHAVIOUR & ACTIVITIES

| | | | | | | |
|---|---|---|---|---|---|---|
| USUAL ENTERING AND EXITING ACTIVITY? | | | | | | |
| CALM BEHAVIOUR WHEN OPENING HIVE? | | | | | | |
| BEES BRINGING POLLEN INTO HIVE? | | | | | | |
| SIGNS OF ROBBERY AMONG THE BEES? | | | | | | |

## HEALTH STATUS

| | | | | | | |
|---|---|---|---|---|---|---|
| BEES SEEM WEAK OR LAZY? | | | | | | |
| HIGH AMOUNT OF DEAD BEES? | | | | | | |
| QUEEN BEE IS PRESENT / IDENTIFIABLE? | | | | | | |
| INFESTATION BY ANTS / ANTS PRESENT? | | | | | | |
| INFESTATION BY WAX MOTH / WAX MOTH PRESENT? | | | | | | |
| NEGATIVE ODOUR NOTICEABLE? | | | | | | |

| COLONY NAME | |
|---|---|
| DATE | |
| TIME | |

## WEATHER CONDITIONS

🌡 _____  ☀ ☁ 🌧 ⛈ ❄
🚩 _____  ☐ ☐ ☐ ☐ ☐

## INSPECTION

| HIVE NUMBER | ① | ② | ③ | ④ | ⑤ | ⑥ |
|---|---|---|---|---|---|---|

## PRODUCTIVITY & REPRODUCTION

| | | | | | | |
|---|---|---|---|---|---|---|
| AMOUNT OF HONEY | | | | | | |
| GENERAL POPULATION | | | | | | |
| AMOUNT OF BROOD | | | | | | |
| AMOUNT OF SPACE | | | | | | |

## BEHAVIOUR & ACTIVITIES

| | | | | | | |
|---|---|---|---|---|---|---|
| USUAL ENTERING AND EXITING ACTIVITY? | | | | | | |
| CALM BEHAVIOUR WHEN OPENING HIVE? | | | | | | |
| BEES BRINGING POLLEN INTO HIVE? | | | | | | |
| SIGNS OF ROBBERY AMONG THE BEES? | | | | | | |

## HEALTH STATUS

| | | | | | | |
|---|---|---|---|---|---|---|
| BEES SEEM WEAK OR LAZY? | | | | | | |
| HIGH AMOUNT OF DEAD BEES? | | | | | | |
| QUEEN BEE IS PRESENT / IDENTIFIABLE? | | | | | | |
| INFESTATION BY ANTS / ANTS PRESENT? | | | | | | |
| INFESTATION BY WAX MOTH / WAX MOTH PRESENT? | | | | | | |
| NEGATIVE ODOUR NOTICEABLE? | | | | | | |

| COLONY NAME | | WEATHER CONDITIONS | | | | | |
|---|---|---|---|---|---|---|---|
| DATE | | 🌡 ___ | ☀ | ⛅ | 🌧 | ⛈ | ❄ |
| TIME | | 🚩 ___ | ☐ | ☐ | ☐ | ☐ | ☐ |

## INSPECTION

| HIVE NUMBER | ① | ② | ③ | ④ | ⑤ | ⑥ |
|---|---|---|---|---|---|---|

## PRODUCTIVITY & REPRODUCTION

| | 1 | 2 | 3 | 4 | 5 | 6 |
|---|---|---|---|---|---|---|
| AMOUNT OF HONEY | | | | | | |
| GENERAL POPULATION | | | | | | |
| AMOUNT OF BROOD | | | | | | |
| AMOUNT OF SPACE | | | | | | |

## BEHAVIOUR & ACTIVITIES

| | 1 | 2 | 3 | 4 | 5 | 6 |
|---|---|---|---|---|---|---|
| USUAL ENTERING AND EXITING ACTIVITY? | | | | | | |
| CALM BEHAVIOUR WHEN OPENING HIVE? | | | | | | |
| BEES BRINGING POLLEN INTO HIVE? | | | | | | |
| SIGNS OF ROBBERY AMONG THE BEES? | | | | | | |

## HEALTH STATUS

| | 1 | 2 | 3 | 4 | 5 | 6 |
|---|---|---|---|---|---|---|
| BEES SEEM WEAK OR LAZY? | | | | | | |
| HIGH AMOUNT OF DEAD BEES? | | | | | | |
| QUEEN BEE IS PRESENT / IDENTIFIABLE? | | | | | | |
| INFESTATION BY ANTS / ANTS PRESENT? | | | | | | |
| INFESTATION BY WAX MOTH / WAX MOTH PRESENT? | | | | | | |
| NEGATIVE ODOUR NOTICEABLE? | | | | | | |

| COLONY NAME | |
|---|---|
| DATE | |
| TIME | |

## WEATHER CONDITIONS

| 🌡️ | ___ | ☀️ ☁️ 🌧️ ⛈️ ❄️ |
|---|---|---|
| 🚩 | ___ | ☐ ☐ ☐ ☐ ☐ |

## INSPECTION

| HIVE NUMBER | ① | ② | ③ | ④ | ⑤ | ⑥ |
|---|---|---|---|---|---|---|

## PRODUCTIVITY & REPRODUCTION

| | | | | | | |
|---|---|---|---|---|---|---|
| AMOUNT OF HONEY | | | | | | |
| GENERAL POPULATION | | | | | | |
| AMOUNT OF BROOD | | | | | | |
| AMOUNT OF SPACE | | | | | | |

## BEHAVIOUR & ACTIVITIES

| | | | | | | |
|---|---|---|---|---|---|---|
| USUAL ENTERING AND EXITING ACTIVITY? | | | | | | |
| CALM BEHAVIOUR WHEN OPENING HIVE? | | | | | | |
| BEES BRINGING POLLEN INTO HIVE? | | | | | | |
| SIGNS OF ROBBERY AMONG THE BEES? | | | | | | |

## HEALTH STATUS

| | | | | | | |
|---|---|---|---|---|---|---|
| BEES SEEM WEAK OR LAZY? | | | | | | |
| HIGH AMOUNT OF DEAD BEES? | | | | | | |
| QUEEN BEE IS PRESENT / IDENTIFIABLE? | | | | | | |
| INFESTATION BY ANTS / ANTS PRESENT? | | | | | | |
| INFESTATION BY WAX MOTH / WAX MOTH PRESENT? | | | | | | |
| NEGATIVE ODOUR NOTICEABLE? | | | | | | |

www.ingramcontent.com/pod-product-compliance
Lightning Source LLC
Chambersburg PA
CBHW080215040426
42333CB00044B/2693